The Pink Identity

My Sessions with a lesbian
a real story

Nncclanjana

Vitasta

Vitasta Publishing Pvt. Ltd.
New Delhi

Published by
Renu Kaul Verma for
Vitasta Publishing Pvt. Ltd.
2/15, Ansari Road, Daryaganj,
New Delhi - 110 002

ISBN 978-93-80828-18-3

A true story. Names of characters changed to respect confidentiality.

Cover Design and Layout by Vitasta Publishing Pvt. Ltd.
Printed by Vits Press, New Delhi

Preface

The sweetest moments of life are lost before we realize
The feeling of pain lingers longer than we recognize.
Life is like a piece of pearl, Hold its beauty, never let it fall

Emotions—we all possess them, but often forget to acknowledge. Are emotions truly a reflection of our mind?

When hurt, a child cries, irrespective of the place, situation or environment. Our social norms teach 'him' to overcome such weak emotions by suppressing or consciously forgetting the pain, while for 'her', the crying is well accepted as a natural occurrence.

When children play together, they fight, cry or laugh without inhibitions, often unaware of their sex or other social, racial and cultural differences. The same groups of friends, in course of time, become 'them' and 'us,' largely influenced by these differences. Among the many prevalent, gender difference is one of the major segregating factors that decide the way boys and girls 'should' behave. Teenage, which is the most delicate and utterly confusing age, is the time when attraction towards the opposite sex first begins. We take it for granted that boys get attracted towards girls and vice-versa.

The problem arises when one comes across those who are attracted to the same sex or for that matter, to both sexes. This is where difference in emotions, behaviours and attitudes surface. Emotions cluster up to play the devil's advocate both ways. Only those who undergo such a dilemma understand what it is to be neither 'them' nor 'us'.

It is from there that the struggle begins. Denial or any form of resistance first surfaces between the 'superficial or imagined self' and the 'real self'. Once that begins to somewhat resolve, dissonance shoots up between 'self' and 'others', who would be the heterosexuals. From here on, starts all the conflicts and differences of opinion among family and friends, if orientation is disclosed. The society as a whole, so to speak, gets involved in the issue. Thus, a homosexual individual often ends up losing self-confidence resulting in an identity crisis, or other forms of insecurities. All these feelings and the process of becoming, what others perceive of him or her, are essentially interplay of emotions which are such that they can make or break relationships, in this context.

Is this true then, that to mature or be treated with respect one must conceal one's emotions? Why is an adult's vulnerability unacceptable? Why is one ridiculed when one does not fit with the trend, or does not conform to accepted norms? Why do we fear to show our real feelings?

The world around us is replete with superficial façades, glamour and fame, such that our childlike unadulterated self often takes a backseat. Despite all external distractions, there is always room for connecting with our true selves. Once we overcome denying our emotions, there is no looking back; rather they allow us to discover, accept, love and learn about who we really are. Once we are able to do this, we become more sensitive and respectful towards others' emotional needs as well.

I consider counselling as a means to connect with one's deepest, even forgotten or suppressed emotions. My experience as a counsellor has done wonders in the way I now understand the process of counselling and healing. It has enabled me to unlock a whole new world of meaningful existence, especially in relationships.

This book is a reminiscence of my experiences as a budding counsellor which are close to my heart and have moulded me to become the person I am today. It is also the story of one of my clients, with whom I shared an unforgettable bond and her struggles and the process to gain respect and self-acceptance as a lesbian. Readers, who have never been exposed to counselling, would get an insight to the process of counselling and its power to heal. All characters in the book are real people but their true identities have been concealed to protect their privacy. This book is based solely on personal experiences and hence no specific community has been targeted.

I hope to reach out to all those who have had similar experiences and also to everyone who would understand the various shades of life with sensitivity.

Witnessing life with a different eye.........

To The Reader

To recognize, to accept, to believe, to confront, to transform and to sustain; means to grow

Celebration of the simple pleasures of life, which we often take for granted, actually adds value to our everyday existence. My journey as a counsellor has not been a bed of roses though it fortified me to understand relationships better. I recognized the value of attentive listening, which had the potential to connect or feel without having to actually live the other's life.

Counselling is all about "clients" and is not a two-way friendly dialogue. This is what naturally differentiates a counsellor from a well-wisher! It is often debated as to what extent client-counsellor relationship should be extended. It is a one-sided power equation where only the client discloses his or her deepest concerns and secrets and the counsellor acts as a blank canvas on which emotions are protrayed. The counsellor's empathetic and unconditional support enables the clients to unlock their inner world. The pace and extent of healing is contingent upon the depth of involvement between the client and the counsellor. Since every client is unique, they present the counsellor with an unmatched set of situations and a new world to explore.

The counsellor needs to attend to the client's world impartially, without being influenced by preconceived notions. Though professionally counsellors are non-judgmental and foreclose their own emotions during sessions- they also desire, feel, love, cry and hate just as everyone else.

My client in this book was one of my first clients, who seemed quite unsettled, rooted deeply within the clutches of everyday hustle bustle. I found her to be quite enlightening in non-traditional ways. Though she seldom shared any optimistic thoughts, I continually realized her unhindered faith to succeed through all odds, beneath her negatives. Michele inspired me to learn more, with each succeeding session that I sat with her.

Michele's life, hopes and desires; her enchanting presence as a client, responsiveness and struggle to overcome; inspired me to write about her.

Although we were different, our differences invited an excellent cultural amalgamation, characterized with a personal touch within the periphery of professionalism.

This is not a work of fiction; it is a real experience. The book touches upon similar moments, situations that many of you might have experienced. It is about the truth of a girl who finds peace after going through an agonising period of denying her reality.

'An attachment between two very dissimilar people, related professionally, who shared, interpreted, cried, laughed, and learned to rejoice life, the way it moulded them.'

Acknowledgements

I dedicate this book to my parents for their unconditional support throughout and for always motivating me to the fullest.

My heartfelt appreciation goes to Mr J K Satyarthi, without whom I could not have written this book. Thank you for sustaining my spirit throughout my journey of writing.

Also, I sincerely thank my clients for believing in me and trusting in therapy. Last but not the least; I thank the entire team of Vitasta Publishing, especially the Publishing Director, Ms Renu Kaul Verma, and my editors for the success of this book.

Contents

Welcome to My World

Change is inevitable;
acceptance of it is beautiful

It has been almost five years since I first met her. The memories, however, are as fresh as though it happened yesterday. I remember my first day of internship at the Counselling Centre of Simmons College, Boston—a gateway to a whole new world.

It was a gloomy day and the absence of the gleaming sun made it seem like evening. My heart was pounding so loudly, I thought everyone in the room could hear it. A classmate of mine and I reached earlier than our allotted time as did the other three interns from the Northeastern College.

Simmons was predominantly a girls' college though co-ed for Master's degree, a renowned institution with a formidable reputation for academic excellence.

We waited in the aesthetically-designed semi-circular room, covered with an earthy brown rug, which camouflaged the wooden floors. Soon, the empty chairs which were arranged in a circle were filled up. The room, initially quiet, had a soft drone of voices. The interns were seated as instructed. Two of the staff members seemed familiar; I recalled them as my interviewers. The seating arrangement was quite unusual from the conventional conference table meetings.

Dr John, the only male staff member, was also the director of the Counselling Centre. This was quite an interesting feature! He was middle-aged, bald with mildly-tanned skin and his rimless glasses glistened when the weak sunlight trickling through the side windows fell on them. Seated on his left was an elderly lady, dressed elegantly in a double-breasted pink coat and white trousers with flat-heeled tan-coloured shoes. She sat with her legs crossed; her thighs and calves seemingly had a negligible difference in shape. This was Dr Sparks, the Head Psychologist and the direct supervisor of all the interns. I found her to be very articulate as she began her speech and perceived her to be pretty approachable. Dr Sparks went through our names in the same order in which we were sitting, after completing her own introduction. It felt like school. Sandra Ettinger was another psychologist and a staff member assigned to assist the interns during group supervision. She was quite young, not very tall, with shiny curly hair and prominent Hispanic features. She, along with Dr Diana, the psychiatrist of the centre, spoke in conjunction about the principle rules and practical approaches regarding the treatment plans. They enumerated the programmes focussing on women's empowerment; some were even featured on their website and college magazine.

Previously during my visit to Simmons, for the initial interview, I had flipped through the pages of their magazine which had such events listed. They sounded interesting–provided one had ample time to invest, certainly an exaggerated expectation from us interns.

All of us were new and began grasping the centre's goals as much as possible, like a sponge in water. I was excited to be in another college, different from my own, as a staff member. I wondered if others felt similarly. Though the meeting was held to impart information about their working style, the overall atmosphere was quite friendly and open to discussions. I enjoyed my first day's experience.

I had barely settled in my new workplace when, Rene, the help-desk assistant, handed me the schedule for the week and the list of clients I had to attend to. "Not many breaks!" I thought, glancing at it first.

My finger tips felt numb, as if anesthetized, as I watched my first client enter. I survived my first session successfully, although she intimidated me with her unending cross-questions. It was only during group discussion with Sandra that I felt reasonably better about my first session. Was I nervous? Of course I was! I could almost feel my pulse competing against the second hand of the timepiece that was angled on the side-table of my office. At some point of time I thought, I did not know what to expect from real clients although the satisfaction of dealing with real clients was unparallelled; pseudo sessions seemed like child's play now. However, the anxiety did not overwhelm my excitement, since I had been waiting eagerly for this time ever since my admission to the post-graduate programme in Boston College.

I soon became accustomed to the continuous influx of clients, as one session followed another, that it no longer felt like the first day! Totally engrossed; I already belonged to the centre. As I waited for my fifth and final client, Michele, I was ready to call it a day as I had reached saturation point by then.

Before Michele's session I had already visited clients back-to-back since noon. The faces, concerns and surroundings, which were strange hitherto, almost immediately became familiar within a single day.

I seconded her name once more from the record sheet, which was filled by the clients themselves at the time of registration. I glanced through her presenting problem, medical history, department, year and so forth. Michele's record sheet looked something like this:

Name: Michele Hobbes

Year: Sophomore

Department: School of Arts, major - nursing

Presenting problems: Feel the need to talk to someone, lonely and depressed at times. I am confused about my sexual preferences and wish to get clarity on that. I often lack confidence and feel low about myself. Relationship with parents is quite disturbing.

Significant medical history: My mother and grandmother are diabetic. I guess it runs in the family!

Referral: Self

Did you visit the Counselling Centre in the last semester? Yes

****

It was five minutes past 3 pm, but there was no sign of my client. The centre had instructed us to wait for a maximum of 15 minutes for a client. I found myself glancing at the clock every couple of seconds.

As I sat, occupied with multiple thoughts, I heard the slightest knock on the loosely-shut door. It was Rene informing me about Michele, who was waiting in the lobby.

We finally settled for our first session at 3:20 pm She immediately apologized, on entering, for her late arrival. Our chairs were placed approximately four feet away, which allowed me to observe my client's posture as we spoke.

This was a bit odd, but I had grown accustomed from the previous sessions to introduce myself in capacity of being their new counsellor, with details of my qualifications in case, they were skeptical about it. I omitted that part of my introduction regarding my Asian origin since it was obvious. Besides my educational information I didn't share further information, maybe I was too conscious. During our conversation it seemed Michele became reasonably comfortable and responded frequently by nodding her head when I spoke. Following the preliminary rapport formation, Michele began narrating her life in bits and pieces, as much she could, to me, a stranger.

11 July, 2003

Session: 1

Her first words, "It's unusual that now I'll be seeing someone different this semester. Previously Lisa was my counsellor and she was great. It's strange not to see her around; I remember we used to meet in this very room."

I certainly felt a bit awkward, not knowing how to react. This was the first time any client discussed her previous counsellor with me. I simply added, "It seems you are missing Lisa."

Michele agreed instantly, "Yeah! I think that's right! I never thought I would. Ever since I had visited this room it was always her and now...." There was a momentary silence. I heard her voice trail away as she looked at me and smiled hesitantly.

I inquired further, "Is change hard?"

Her response was quick, "Well! You know I think it is, especially when the change is unknown but we do grow accustomed to it. Initially when I had started with Lisa, it took me some time to open up and be myself. This time, it feels a bit easier with you."

My mind speculated on how hard it must be for her.

In the next couple of minutes only silence spoke as we listened to our thoughts I observed that whenever she spoke it was more about Lisa than herself.

"I don't have one specific thing to discuss.. There are some issues that disturb me, especially my relationship with my parents," she said breaking the silence.

I responded optimistically, "I am glad you are comfortable sharing your immediate concerns."

Michele continued gazing far away at the window behind me, "I don't know where to start, and it's all so interrelated. Sometimes I find it hard to verbalize my thoughts coherently. Do you think this is unusual?"

"No, not at all, it happens to all of us at some time or the other," I reassured her. I added, "All means of communication are open to you, if writing works better to start with, go for it."

She smiled and thanked me. Then hesitantly added, "Actually Lisa encouraged me to pen down my thoughts and it worked, so I was thinking …if it would be okay to….”

I interrupted, “Certainly! Whatever floats your boat I'm fine with it, as long as we communicate.”

As the clock was ticking away, I briefed her that only a last couple of minutes were left for the session to end. I wondered if there would be flurry of any last-minute details before leaving, as had happened with two of my previous clients. However, Michele did not do so. Instead she ended our first session confessing that she felt a bit awkward accepting someone else in Lisa's place. I appreciated her truth as much as her silence and hesitation to open up with me.

****

The following Monday I had an early supervision with Dr Audrey Sparks. Being the senior psychologist at the centre, she seemed to me to be the best mentor to solve queries. Dr Sparks' demeanour as well as her appearance often reminded me of my grandmother, of whom I was rather fond.

My first supervision went better than expected; better than my sessions actually. We started with a couple of initial housekeeping concerns, namely, scheduling the list of ongoing clients with Rene, having information about the appropriate workshops offered in case the clients inquired, dealing with clients who missed their appointments and a few other paper-work formalities. I found Dr Sparks to be pretty approachable and friendly.

We discussed my tough luck with the first client and how I recovered with other clients in the later sessions. Initially, I had been nervous attending my first client's aggressive questioning but gradually I was able to see and think beyond my own diffidence.

Interestingly, among all clients I had met so far, Michele fascinated me the most, though I felt a sense of inaptness during sessions with her. I spoke more about her; as compared to my other clients during supervision, a point that Dr Sparks noticed. While I narrated Michele's longing for Lisa, she inquired if Michele was sad while remembering Lisa, to which I agreed.

It was challenging to be compared with another counsellor. I thought aloud with Dr Sparks that this might not work since it would be quite painful for Michele to reconnect. She agreed, but also reminded me that it was only the first session and too early to draw conclusions. At the end of the session, I confided that this was nothing like what I had experienced before, in all the pseudo sessions during my practical classes.

In conclusion, Dr Sparks said, "Beginnings are often hard to manage and it takes time to settle. Also, a strong bond with clients would imbibe all hesitations and allow transparency within the counselling relationships."

I knew she was right. She further enlightened, "You'll see how practical experiences will facilitate your professional growth as a counsellor. Therapy, in turn, will open avenues for introspection, the most fascinating aspect of therapy. The journey has only just begun; be informed and alert about your own feelings as much as you are about your clients."

Passing through the convenient stores and the mall entrance that evening, situated next to the train-station on The Fenway, my mind raced back to the day's events. I felt exhilarated.

I thought to myself, "I did it! I deliberated upon my first client, Amy, and her pressing concern over her figure and her unending longing for desirable attention from the oppositie sex. Though she seemed healthy overall, her diet merely consisted of diet coke and diet chips. There was lot to explore about Amy in the coming sessions."

The crowd inside the train was unaware of my new-found world and my achievements. Slowly the rhythm of the train's movement lulled my thoughts and brought me back to the mundane world. I was seated next to a young American couple, busy sharing their sweet nothings. It reminded me of my college days. I thought of Sasndy and Shwets, as we referred them, who were the only two dating then, within our group of five. Their dates often remained the hot topic during off periods.

It is true that the feelings of love and attraction are the same across culture, only the expression changes. In US, it ws not unusual to catch glimpse of couples kissing in public, even gay couples for that matter. I was absorbing all of it like a sponge and actually enjoying the openness of expressions in the US.

****

The week went by very soon, most days I shuttled between Simmons Counselling Centre and Boston College to attend my classes; thus travelling swallowed a major chunk of my time. It was a hectic schedule: mornings essentially consisted of endless group meetings followed by sessions later in the day and then evening classes at Boston College.

The majority of my clients were Caucasian women between

the age group of 18 and 22 years. Depression, homesickness, culture-shock, drug/alcohol abuse, peer pressure, and betrayal in relationships were the common agendas. Some did have rather serious issues or pre-existing medical conditions that demanded special psychiatric attention. I was learning in multitudes, the exhaustion was undoubtedly a part of the package.

Soon I realized that the train station had transformed into my resting and snacking junction. Initially, I would return home with anxieties and worries, a carry-over from the sessions, but that changed with time as I learned to detach myself from the process, an essential lesson for counsellors. Although the process was exhausting, it was intrinsically satisfying too. I would always be fascinated that within minutes of stepping inside the room, my clients would cease to be strangers and I would be privy to their deepest secrets and wrenching sorrows. The astounding power of therapy left me speechless, every time I ended a session.

18 July, 2003

Session: 2

On Friday around 3 pm, the centre was almost deserted. Most of my fellow interns had left early owing to cancellations. I had just commenced updating my records when Michele walked in. This time she was on time. We warmed up by discussing general topics. This made her feel at ease. Michele spoke about her stress and concerns about time-management in her nursing programme. In course of the conversation, she revealed her desire to identify her individuality, as one of the foremost reasons for pursuing counselling.

Individuality! The word demanded my extra attention as she uttered it. I wanted her to speak a bit more on that. However, she switched the topic.

Michele's blue eyes were packed with questions, which she could not answer. I also noticed her choice of attire and fondness for bright colours. Michele's blonde hair was loosely done in a pony tail, cascading down her shoulders. Her silver nose ring complimented her features well. She looked Italian by origin. I learned of Michele's love for ethnic jewellery from the earrings and bracelets she wore. I wondered if she was aware of the Indian ethnic jewellery.

My thoughts were interrupted by her voice, "You know, it's all so interrelated, feels kind of odd to reiterate what I had already once narrated to Lisa but I'll try."

I calmly looked at her and smiled at her remark. There was a momentary silence.

She began, "I'd like to talk about my family first, since that is where it all started. My little sister Emily and I are very close. She is the only one in my family with whom I can share. I don't know what to say next...."

Michele began gazing at the floor, I urged, "It seems you really love your sister and trust her too."

"Hmm...that's true. She is the only one in whom I can confide. It has been two years since I have been away from home in Simmons. In these past months I have dated many people, which only Emily is aware of. Commitment is hard for me, which is why my previous two relationships broke down," she ended.

I clarified, "You find it hard to sustain long-term relationships, right? Could you elaborate a bit more on that?"

"Yes", she stated, "It's like... like... I sometimes feel unsure if I really like or still find my partner as attractive as I did in the beginning. I also tend to get attracted to both sexes and that's frustrating because I don't understand if my attraction is for real or not. Does this make sense to you?," she asked, narrowing her eyes.

"Of course it does," I assured, "Also I'm not here to judge you for right or wrong. Whatever happens in this room stays in this room. Maybe I'm wrong and correct me if so, but it sounds like you are unsure about your sexual orientation."

Michele readily agreed and mentioned that it was rather becoming her sole concern lately.

Following a brief pause she said, "It was really comforting to hear you address this before I mentioned it since you belong to a different culture."

A bell rang inside my head! While I was trying to make sense of her views, Michele continued and interrupted my thoughts.

She continued, "So, like I was telling you...my attraction towards both the sexes has created a lot of confusion lately. Darren was my first serious relationship; we were good friends in junior high. Our friendship grew intimate and I enjoyed the intimacy and the passionate love he endowed me with. Unfortunately, our relationship was short-lived and I soon broke up. I thought I loved him as much as he did, but it turned out to be a different story."

I questioned in between, "Do you regret losing him?"

Michele looked at me, seemingly recollecting her past memories, "We dated for three months but soon my mind began wandering towards others. You know, I felt like a jerk feeling this way! There had been instances when I had the urge to sleep with other guys, while dating Darren. All this eventually soured our relationship, but I never felt sad. Instead, I loved my sovereignty to date whoever I wished, once we got separated."

I clarified, "Seems like committing to one was becoming stressful and you were happy to break free."

"Yeah, it was as if I was hiding my own liberty while I was with them. Weeks later, Darren offered to patch up if I 'behaved', she explained by lifting the first two fingers of her both hands to mention "behaved" within quotes.

"I was happy being single, enjoying life my way. I dated off and on, some on a friendly note and some out of infatuation. It was all fun! Emily was the only one who knew about my sporadic sexual encounters."

It was our second session and she hadn't mentioned Lisa or her reaction even once. This could work, I thought, since we both were trying to connect.

I reminded Michele, peeping at my watch, that the session was coming to an end. In the last couple of minutes, she had relaxed and was slowly sipping from her water bottle in between dialogues. Her openness and body language explicitly indicated the comfort level, which Michele later affirmed verbally as well. I scheduled her for next week, same time, while she packed her bottle inside her suede burgundy-coloured bag.

Her session was the last one for the day and also for the week. I bade Rene goodbye and left the space, which I referred to myself as "The world of free minds."

The cool breeze outside refreshed me and lessened my fatigue as I headed towards the train station. July was indeed pleasant in Boston, unlike Delhi. Post-sunset, the evenings became even more exciting, especially, with the approaching weekend.

My classes at Boston College generally continued late, stretching until 10 pm. Sadly enough, such schedules did not render me the opportunity to enjoy the beautiful amber-glazed sunsets except on Fridays and weekends. Meals too were on way while commuting from Simmons to college. Due to time constraints, we seldom ventured to dine out and mostly ate at the college cafeteria. The dining halls partially filled up after the evening classes. Often I had my dinner there because it got too late to eat after reaching home.

The cafeteria was the most happening place in the college, the constant influx of undergraduate/graduate students filled up the place with laughter, frolic and fun. The food, undoubtedly, was delicious, considering my Indian palate. My all-time favourite was macaroni with mixed greens and sautéed broccoli on the side. Besides excellent pita bread, wholewheat grilled sandwiches, chicken/pork/fish roll and an unending platter of sushi and salads were also served to tempt the palate. The unending platter of desserts ranged from the choicest of icecreams to the most sophisticated *crépe suzettes*. Nonetheless, there was nothing compared to a home-cooked meal.

****

Saturday, 5 am

I had woken up earlier than usual, refreshed from last night's extended sleep. The morning walk made it even better! It was cool and windy outside. Many strolled with their pets around the riverside park which included a serene pond surrounded by lush greens. The blue and green together attracted walkers from all around the neighbourhood.

My refreshed mind was all ready to start the day, beginning with writing the process notes for my clients. (Process notes were my own reflections about the clients during the sessions.)

This is what I wrote for Michele:

There was slight hesitation while Michele spoke in her first two sessions, which I thought was quite natural. In between discussions, she remained quiet and sat silently just smiling occasionally. Presumably she was nervous and felt awkward talking about herself at this stage. I knew there were a lot of pent-up emotions trapped inside her mind as Michele expressed herself.

There was certainly some indecisiveness about her sexual orientation. Her dating experiences had left her confused. Michele spoke about her desire to ascertain her individuality as one of the prime reasons for therapy. I wondered what she exactly meant. She made an interesting remark about me, belonging from a different culture. Her comment made me wonder if it were a reflection of her curiosity towards my culture. I pondered over what she thought of me, as an Indian, as a woman of colour. Her words made me curious about her latent thoughts regarding me, my culture and so forth.

I understand it is hard for Michele to reconnect with someone else as a counsellor that easily. We need to talk about this probably in one of the sessions. Time, time and more time was the only solution to make it work.

I Learn to Discover

Trust your instincts;
they never betray you

The weekend went by in a jiffy and I had just enough time to finish all the pending work. Monday morning—sitting in room 2B in front of the computer—I began chalking out all the meetings and appointments for the day while waiting for my supervision.

I anticipated this supervision to bring forth insightful thoughts about Michele besides my other queries. It was fascinating to notice the level of personal interest that was beginning to surface with this client, of which I gradually became well aware. I wanted to understand my own development process as a counsellor and why I found Michele so fascinating. I had no clear idea what led me to think of her so often in just two sessions. I was clueless. Maybe I just simply liked her or it could be because she was the first one to compare me with another counsellor. At the back of my mind I knew Michele had dated women also, maybe that was intimidating for me to accept. Although I was mostly attracted to tall, dark and handsome men, dating the same-sex wasn't wrong for me but yes it was different. A matter of choice probably, but I had to come to terms with it to accept it easily.

Dr Sparks, probably, was the right person to provide some answers to my dilemma.

The day was loaded with a profuse list of new and existing clients, which I attended subsequent to my supervision. Back-to-back sessions, limitless paper work, introduction with new clients—time just flew! Through the week, I felt my life was beginning to be governed by clients! The experiences my clients extracted out of me, my deepest thoughts, unknown responses, anticipations and fears, unexpected moments of silence and jubilation, everything seemed so intense. I felt as if I was discovering myself afresh in the course of understanding them. Each day was a rollercoaster ride of emotions.

Since I belonged to a different culture with an unfamiliar accent and distinct looks, many clients reacted rather cautiously towards me initially. They inquired about my nationality but refrained from commenting much, probably owing to their trivial knowledge about Indians. I was pleasantly surprised when one of my Irish clients actually spoke to me in broken Hindi forming simple easy sentences. She was a student of foreign studies and had opted India as her choice of study. Beth came across as a sweet soft-spoken person. She was homesick since all of her family was in Scotland. It took me some time to understand her native accent while she spoke to me in English. She regretted leaving her boyfriend back home for her higher studies. Interesting client but she seemed overanxious. Many students preferred Asian counsellors; since I was the only one among all the interns, I got quite a colourful range of clients. However, my Indian clients did not make any concessions and were among the toughest.

Rupa was one of them who constantly speculated about my thoughts to the extent that she even inquired if I ever felt judgmental or criticized her after the sessions. It was frustrating to sit through such baseless curiosity and suspicion. My other Indian client was no better either! Sheba continually presented new weekly issues, deferring from disclosing the truth in the previous sessions. I felt there wasn't any genuine problem except for her nagging behaviour for each and every little thing.

It seemed because of the strong family bonds and the tradition of "keeping it within the family" in Indian society counsellors were "outsiders" rather than professional helpers. Sometimes Asian clients evaluated my professional competence by bringing up topics which were at cross-purposes. Although it would be unfair to draw inferences from a handful of clients, they reflected the skepticism and taboo towards counselling within the Asian community. On the contrary, most of my Caucasian clients trusted more and disclosed uninhibitedly which could have been due to the cultural openness in the West.

In the midst of such experiences, Dr Sparks guided me like a true mentor. She supported me through all such situations, tricky uncanny questions and my dilemmas. She taught me to sit "big" on the counsellor's chair without making the client feel inferior. Before my internship, I had not known about the role of power between the client-counsellor relationship, but I managed to learn over a period of time. Once Dr Sparks had lightly commented that perhaps due to my petite figure, many of the clients denied me my position or felt I was too naïve to handle their vulnerabilities. It makes me laugh now when I think of it, but maybe it was true. I did encounter some very tough clients during the first couple of months.

I found that self-discovery was the most fascinating part of the therapy. Many a time I discovered traits about myself in the presence of Dr Sparks, as did my clients while with me. It was like a light bulb being switched on inside my mind. Besides personal enhancement, I taught myself to feel worthy for what I was assigned and convey the same to my clients. I realized that to be accepted by clients, I had to prove myself professionally. I had to let go off the thinking of being accepted merely because of my qualifications.

With Sherri Ettinger, our group supervisor, we often discussed topics related to culture and therapy where Celina, a Turkish ex-intern, and I added to the multi-cultural perspective of the discussions. It was insightful to know how clients might envision cultural disparity and the potential impact of it on counselling.

Except for Michele, I needed to prove my credentials to almost all my clients. Interestingly, there were no issues about who exercised more power or any sort of professional cross-questioning while I was in session with Michele. I remember in one of the supervisions, while discussing Michele, Dr Sparks had remarked, "You seem to be truly engrossed with this client."

My concern had escalated when she vented her doubts regarding desirability for both sexes; unknowingly I became a bit conscious of my own thoughts. I suppose belonging to a culture where sexual orientation is mostly taken for granted as being male or female, it took me a while before I could accept beyond the obvious. I was unsure if Michele sensed my hesitation on the topic. However, she did mention feeling comfortable discussing her sexual preferences in session, which meant she was unaware of my awkwardness.

I spoke with Dr Sparks if it were any good to discuss the dynamics of our relationship since Michele had already touched upon it indirectly. Perhaps exploring our differences might allow me to understand Michele better because we could be more transparent about what to expect from counselling.

To Dr Sparks, perhaps, it came as an everyday inquiry, I wondered if other interns also struggled through similar issues. She discussed about the importance of the client and the counsellor's relationship and unconditional acceptance of the clients.

"Exploring mutual relationship is often helpful as it can fetch you clarity," Dr. Sparks remarked. Her smile conveyed the faith she vested in me, which was very encouraging.

It was Dr Sparks' insight that finally urged me to discuss our relationship with Michele and any cultural hindrances that could impede counselling. I knew this was a move in the right direction. Though there was an element of fear, I feared what if Michele did not entertain such conversations? However, the process had the potential to deliver transparency in our mutual understanding, which could be beneficial in the later sessions. In my position as a counsellor, I had more power to actually navigate our conversation accordingly, but then my conscience forbade me to force the topic. I wanted it to be a natural process. The night before the session, I framed a million ways to introduce the topic about discussing our mutual feelings, but none seemed good enough. The night seemed to have halted my thoughts and I accepted it as a well-deserved break, until the actual time approached.

Friday, the day before the weekend, was the day when we were allowed to wear casuals and that itself lessened our stress. At 3 pm when it was time for Michele's arrival, I thought she had no idea how much time I was devoting to her lately. She entered the centre 15 minutes early.

25 July, 2003

Session: 3

I initiated the conversation beginning with the dynamics of our relationship. Michele prompted instantly, "You know this is amazing! I too thought about our cultural differences in spite of feeling so comfortable in sessions."

I appreciated her eagerness and encouraged her to share her opinion uninhibitedly.

Michele willingly nodded, "Sure! You know, Lisa did this activity as well, so I am a bit accustomed to it. It was great to have Lisa as my counsellor and I hope that it'll work just as well with you too. This room feels very comforting to me; it acts like a safety blanket. I feel I'm heard and accepted for who I am," and added smilingly, "It'll be interesting to see an Asian counsellor this year."

In response to her thoughts I explained, "Sometimes I might think differently; we all do— be it cultural or individual opinion, but I would truly appreciate if you address any such thoughts that might disturb you. Always feel free to communicate whatever you wish to."

Following this, Michele insisted on starting from where she had left the previous session. Michele recounted her teenage years, "Those numerous relationships during high school did not excite me much, although I was always seeing someone. I switched from one to another partner frequently, and tried to fit in my peer group. Initially, I did get attracted, but later it felt pointless to continue with the same person."

Further, she clarified that the relationships were with both the sexes. I urged Michele to elaborate on her expectations from a relationship.

She replied, "During high school I was unsure about what I really wanted. Hanging out with boys helped one to fit in and so I did! I guess that's quite a shallow thing to do. However, Simmons changed my outlook."

I interrupted, "So it was during high school that you started getting attracted towards both sexes?"

"Exactly, I was coming to that part. My experience at Simmons College was nothing like before. The first semester offered immense changes, internal as well as external. Leaving home was not as bad as I had expected. Rather, I celebrated my freedom by exchanging emails and letters with Emily. My parents, of course, were unaware of all my dating stuff."

"At Simmons, I became clearer and more aware of my feelings. During the first semester, I shared an apartment with one of my classmates. She was dating a guy, who often spent nights at our apartment with her. In the beginning things went fine, but soon his visits became more frequent. I found it hard to concentrate on my work without getting distracted by their romantic talk and physical intimacy. My friend and I argued several times but it only made matters worse. Unable to handle the situation, I started spending nights at another friend's place."

"It must have been really hard living this way?," I interrupted.

"I guess I had no choice," Michele sighed, "The rent was cheaper compared to other places. Moreover, I was in the waiting list to get accommodated in the college dorm, so it was a temporary thing."

It surprised me that she was well aware of the passing time even when engrossed so profoundly, ending abruptly as it was almost time to wrap up the session. She ended, "This time is precious but too short; I wait all week for this to talk, express and to feel whatever."

I commented, "Yes it's time for now, but we always have next time, right?"

Michele stood up to straighten her skirt; I noticed it was the same she had worn in the previous session, probably it was her favourite. Later that evening, I thought about Michele's facility with words. As I did so, a thought came to my mind, "Do I speak that well?" I had absolutely no idea why I was comparing myself with her. I tried to analyse my seemingly random thoughts....

Was I jealous?

Was I self-conscious?

Or was I confused, like she was about her dating partners?

With these thoughts whirling in my head, I headed home. There were no classes scheduled on Friday evenings. This allowed me to enjoy the spectacular sunset, which I could not otherwise rest of the week. It was a cherished time in my weekly routine.

Back home, I had just settled down on the sofa and eased off my shoes, when a sudden thought about an assignment made me jump up again. I had to submit it on Monday. I reconfirmed the date in my planner, just in case I was mistaken since I was in no mood to work on something as dry as statistics over the weekend. However, I had no option but to work, post-dinner, that night.

Before hitting the sack, I slipped back to my session with Michele. I was happy and, more so, genuinely relieved that Michele initiated willingly to explore about our mutual differences. I sensed a slight hint of detachment, or even latent anger towards her parents, as she spoke today.

****

Things often felt boring with the same routine everyday. Weekends were fun when I could meet a couple of my friends and enjoy a brunch or go out for shopping. Monday dawned with the promise of a whole new week to chart out new plans and thoughts.

I never missed a chance to observe my surroundings. Off campus as I walked most of the mornings I found lesbian couples holding hands, a few warmly embracing each other's warm touch. Initially I would stare at them wondering how unlikely to imagine something alike so public in India. With time I became more accepting or probably got acclimatized with it.

Most of my Mondays mornings were better off than the rest of the week because of supervision sessions. It always carved out something interesting! While walking through Fenway at 8 am, towards Simmons, that morning, my thoughts were again around Michele. Was this abnormal? Earlier, I was comparing myself to her and now these early morning thoughts!

Why was I thinking only about Michele? Was it an inferiority complex? Was I intimidated because of her bisexual encounters? My thoughts floated like clouds in the sky.

During supervision that morning, I brought forward this concern to Dr Sparks. To begin with, she found it rather amusing. However, on a serious note, she inquired if I felt similarly for any other client. I clarified that I had not and that it was the first time that I ever felt this way. Dr Sparks stared at me through her glasses and smiled softly.

She said reassuringly, "I understand your concern and it's good to be aware and articulate your feelings explicitly. I'd prefer not to give an opinion now, it's too early. Sometimes we become more attached to some clients, which is quite natural. Personal likings, favouritism, partiality, do creep in at times. The wisest thing to do is to keep yourself informed of such internal changes and accept them. There can be layers of explanations for why you feel the way you do. Maybe we could do some counselling sessions exploring your life and reflect on such concerns from there on."

I considered her suggestion for a few minutes. Although I was a bit hesitant and nervous about doing sessions on my personal life, I agreed.

"It might simply inculcate confidence within you," she responded, flipping through a psychoanalysis text. "Your inhibitions can lead to obstacles in therapy, so always accept your thoughts but don't get swayed by them. From my years of experience, I have observed that therapy is at two levels. Level one is an ongoing process that occurs between the client and the counsellor. The second level, which I always find more challenging, is to understand and differentiate between one's personal thoughts and professional thoughts as a counsellor."

I took note of her advice and thanked her. Later I discussed Rupa and Sheba's issue around counselling and their skeptic attitude. Dr. Sparks suggested explaining them in depth about the counselling rule of ethics and assuring them that everything would be kept confidential, repeatedly at every session until they finally start believing in the process. Dr Sparks spoke animatedly, "BINGO!!! I think you answered your problem right there."

Her insightful words made me think long after we had finished the session. She had pointed out the core of therapy, while focussing on the detachment factor from clients. I agreed because it allowed an impartial eye to counsellors, to see things without being restricted by their own prejudices. I understood that we all imbibe certain pre-conceived notions, ideas, and beliefs while growing up and thereafter. However, as a counsellor, it is mandatory to seal those personal preferences within and remain impartial as much as possible and let clients explore their own. For instance, my acceptance of same-sex romantic relationships and empathizing with their feelings never contradicted with my own sexual preferences.

This was one of most meaningful supervisions I had during my internship. Previously, I was embarrassed to accept my underlying thoughts regarding Michele, but later it became quite acceptable. Not only did this concern clarify my hesitations about Michele but also gave me scope to explore my own life during the sessions with Dr Sparks. It facilitated me to reflect on my feelings before beginning to understand clients at depth. My new-found insight about my own thoughts became a major source of exploration as well as inspiration for growing in this profession. During sessions, as Dr Sparks had advised, I remained non-judgmental, as I tried to understand my client's thoughts. Especially with Michele, I visited her world from a counsellor's perspective without interfering with them with my own assumptions. This experience went a long way to help me establish myself professionally. The week had been fanatically busy with just enough time to text message to a few of my loved ones. Was life changing or had I succumbed to my schedule so much that leisure became secondary?

My last client for Thursday evening called to cancel. It had been a while since I had fetched myself an extra hour, though endless things scurried in. I decided to call it a day and leave early. While I was signing out, Rene at the reception informed me about Michele's request for an early appointment at 2 pm, which I confirmed. It was only three in the afternoon; the weather outside was dull and grey. There was a light shower and slight breeze. However, the clouds were piling up, thick and grey, portending a heavy downpour. As the rain fell softly, I walked quickly to the train stop to catch the earliest train.

"Multi-Cultural Issues" was scheduled at 4 pm, a class that always interested me. Luckily, I made it to the class just before it began pouring. There was scant attendance owing to the bad weather. The course helped me to identify aspects from my own life, especially the cultural shock I faced after coming to the US. The class failed to hold my attention for long on that day; I was distracted by various thoughts crowding my mind. I thought about home, I missed speaking to Ma, I thought about the loneliness of old couples living alone, fears and uncertainties of youth and so forth. The topic of discussion in class was bilingualism; only a few fitted that category and I was one of them.

It would have been a far more interesting lecture had I not been so emotionally exhausted.

The evening was dark when the class got over. I headed home, smelling the wetness all around me. The heavy downpour had petered off to a drizzle. The droplets settled on my hair and my trousers were partially wet from walking in the rain. The train station was milling with the evening rush-hour commuters. I managed to get a seat near a window in the crowded train. I looked out and watched the wet stones beneath the overlapping train tracks running beside the shuttle tracks. There was a skimpy layer of mist over the tree tops as the evening sky quietly retired into darkness. I got off at my usual stop and boarded the bus that would take me home. I enjoyed my quiet walk home from the bus stop. The trees, the grass on the pavements, the path, the pebbles which adorned the front entrances of the houses, the fencing— I knew every detail on that path.. The familiarity and the sense of belonging were wonderful. The daily walk home down the tree-lined path was one of the most enjoyable parts of my day.

I unlocked my door and stepped inside. I quickly got out of my wet clothes and took a relaxing shower which rejuvenated my senses. I curled up on the sofa in the living room with a bowl of black bean soup and tossed greens which I had cooked earlier, along with some store-bought *chapattis*. I switched on the television to surf the channels while I ate. There was a lot of work to cover, like always, but I surrendered to the random images flashing on the screen to allow myself to replenish my energy and decided to nap early.

****

Life before Boston

Knowing has no beginning, no end.
It is an ongoing process that evolves,
folds and overlaps

It is a new and unfamiliar experience to write about myself. Nonetheless, I have tried to go beyond the hesitation and inhibitions that might affect the honesty of my narrative. My experiences have shaped me to become the person I am today. Deviating a bit from my life at Boston, here is a snapshot of my life before I started counselling clients and life changed beyond recognition.

We immigrated to the United States in 2002 after I had completed my Bachelor's in Psychology. Until then Delhi was my home and will always be in a way; a place where my childhood memories abound. I had grown up in the warm cocoon of family which had protected me from the rough and tumble of life. In addition to academic and professional growth, the West enabled me to handle a multitude of circumstances independently. It was here that I stepped out to a world of struggles, hopes, dreams, fears, wishes, and limitless possibilities. I became exposed to various cultures, faiths, diverse lifestyles and dialects. This new world was an intricate mosaic of diverse people. It was at times scary, knowing that so much unknown was waiting for me. I thought of myself as a caterpillar coming out of its chrysalis as a butterfly, fluttering wings tentatively in the sun.

Four days after 9/11 marked our advent to the United States. We were one of the few Asians at the Washington airport, owing to the incident, waiting for our connecting flight to Rochester, NY. The experience was nothing like before. I remember noticing each and every detail at the airport, the flawless carpeted floors, the scented air, the clean dust-free chairs, counter tops, the decked-up duty-free shops and cafés, people waiting in queue at the check-in counters, and the restrooms of course; I wondered how could everything be so perfect!

I felt strange looking at myself in the restroom mirror, contrasting against all other white-skinned blondes. As I sat in the waiting area, I observed the crowd; it was amazing to see so many diverse groups of people under one roof. Some had an unusual punk-style of dressing, while some were in formals. There were people from Mexico, China, Europe and India. I heard English being spoken in a variety of accents. I saw a few blonde kids giggling away, displaying their bad teeth! The airport resting areas were filled with the aroma of freshly-brewed coffee, steaks, French croissants and muffins. It was tempting and we gave in and had a quick snack.

I had read articles on racial discrimination and differential treatment given to non-Whites, but to experience it in person was challenging. A store had decorated a display window with some coloured candles along with a cluster of white ones. It looked quite striking; I thought we were much like the coloured candles against all the White people. My father was the only Asian male I could see, and it felt inexplicably strange. Racism, as I understand it today, would have been unknown to me without such personal experience. A few pompous middle-aged blondes with scarlet red nails and fussy hair-dos, scrutinized us with undisguised suspicion, which I thought was quite natural on their part in the context of the 9/11 mishap. My initial experiences at the airport made me realize that we indeed belonged to a very distant world in more than one sense. My experience might sound odd as a lot of Asians do travel to the US frequently, but it was the 9/11 incident which caused such reactions. Had we arrived at a different time perhaps my experience might have been more pleasant.

We stepped outside the Rochester airport which was not that busy as I had expected. Florescent yellow Toyota taxis were lined along the red-brick pavement; most of them had African-American drivers, with a few exceptions. Airconditioned shuttle buses routinely halted at their respective stops and at the mini-traffic signal which was installed to control the airport traffic. It was close to dawn, around 2 am Central Time, if I recall correctly. The lights of the passing vehicles and the streetlights shone translucently through the thin morning mist along the smooth roads.

My watch had two dials, one each for home and world time. Home time showed 1:30 pm; mentally I still had not left India. It was strange to set the US time as home and India as the world time. The sky looked unusually clear without any dust haze; a few stars glistened as though welcoming us. We reached my uncle's house, where we stayed initially. We stayed awake for the rest of the night, partly because of the jet lag and mostly because of the excitement of seeing one another again. Later during the day, unable to resist the temptation of dreaming in a new country, in a new land, in a new bed, I fell asleep.

****

Days followed and so did our destiny to yet another city in Texas. This was Houston, hub of an oil source, located in the south of the US, largely influenced by Mexican inhabitants. Tex-Mex food, Hispanic dialectic and English in a southern accent are quite prevalent. Texas, the Cowboy state, has less natural beauty and more concrete buildings, huge spacious houses, malls and parking lots. I noticed the stiff grass growing along the sidewalks and pavements.

Several nights, as I lay on my bed, I thought wonderingly, "So this is America all about, a place where people come to earn in dollars, where Hollywood becomes real, where the Statue of Liberty poses smartly, where Shahrukh Khan comes to shoot his movies ever so often!"

There were picture-perfect streets which had very few people, parking lots bigger than the departmental stores, miscellaneous colours of hair and skin, unlimited food and equally unlimited wastage of food, shiny broad freeways with cars racing in their respective lanes, the famous Wal-Mart, Macy's and others brands, fast life, and unparalleled public display of love and affection —this was America. One thing that I realized within a week of my arrival in the US was that movies gave a very different picture of what the US really is!

Delhi and Houston being on the same latitude share similar climatic conditions; the days were hot but the central airconditioning systems kept the interiors cool. The evenings were more pleasant in Houston than Delhi, perhaps due to the presence of Galveston beach situated a 100 miles away. During my time in Houston, I worked at a Courtesy Booth for a short while. During this time I picked up bits of Spanish and learnt about the money system in the US and to distinguish between the nickels, dimes, pennies and quarters. I learnt something new everyday! I made a few friends and found Hispanics to be quite down-to-earth and friendly.

Within a few months, I moved to Boston after being enrolled in Boston College for the Master's programme. Boston, I call it the city of intellectuals, was unparalleled for its natural beauty. It was an entirely different city from Houston. Though predominantly White, the presence of international students made the city seem more multi-racial. It was quite like if North Campus in Delhi would transform itself into a city. The charming characteristic feature of Boston was the students, scurrying with their backpacks from one destination to another between the countless colleges and universities, for which the city was famous. Art, dance, theatre, literature and academics formed the heart of Boston. The beautiful surroundings were so inspirational that they could turn analytical brains into a poet's mind. It was a symphony of colours ––with the russet of the maple trees and the myriad shades of green of the oak and evergreens. It was not a city that went to sleep early, primarily because of the large number of students. The pubs, restaurants and discotheques were popular among the young and were quite crowded on the weekends.

Boston had this old-world charm with its amber and red-coloured brick pavements all through the city. The open-air cafés and dinettes were the perfect mood enhancers. I missed being with someone special on such occasions, especially when it snowed. Nature filled the heart with romance and denying its existence would be a sin. I discovered that the city had numerous antique shops. Many of them had thick wooden doors that had copper bells fitted on them which tinkled whenever the doors swung open or shut. They reminded me of the many little Tibetan shops found in hill-stations like Nainital and Manali. I loved the experience of travelling in trains which divided the roads in the middle and ran throughout the city. The sound of the train's bell which went "ting-ting" at every stop reminded me of the trams in Kolkata. It brought back memories of childhood, watching theatre at Rabindrasadan with my grandfather and strolling around Victoria Memorial, and eventually indulging in *jhal muri* or other delicacies or stopping to admire the variety of *sandesh* boxes. I relived those precious moments again in my mind although I was far away both in time and space.

Admission to Boston College opened new avenues and enabled me to explore the vast scope of Psychology, especially counselling. My course in Boston College which was Mental Health Counselling Psychology offered an understanding of the complex human mind through a blend of emotions and culture. The vast expanse of books in the three libraries at the college was more delightful than I had imagined. I initially loved spending time browsing through the books but as my schedule got hectic, I seldom got time to indulge in reading for pleasure. Academically, the course not only guided me towards becoming a professional but also enhanced my sensitivity as a person.

My new friendships and acquaintances consisted of people from almost all over the world. The International Students' Society, of which I became an active member, had members from every country. What a fascinating experience it was to share the world under one roof! In spite of the busy schedule, during the weekends I went out for sightseeing or lunch with friends from the International Students' Society. Not only was it fun interacting with people from across the world but also the Society gave us an opportunity to learn a few words of greeting and a few basic sentences in French, Chinese and Spanish. My classmates, roommates, workmates, interns, friends, clients, and, of course, all my instructors, became my extended family and my life revolved around them. I willingly accepted the change in my life which was to have a lasting effect although it meant that I would be away from home, my parents and old friends.

The tingling coolness outside the centrally-heated homes at the crack of dawn hinted at the soon-to-arrive winter and the nights whispered the same through occasional cold fronts. I became accustomed to the chilly winds which blew in sudden gusts. Being a keen observer of nature, I never missed an opportunity to appreciate it–the multi-coloured fall leaves dangling from branches, the winding pathways and the tall pine trees standing erect. It seemed as if several invisible artists were always at work, painting nature with colours that my eyes had never seen.

The train service, referred to as "T", remained crowded at all times, especially in the morning with officer-goers, teachers, students and other daily passengers. I was required to travel so much that the train became like a second home to me. I started recognising some of the people who used to board the same train with me everyday.

All stops prior to my stop seemed to be the longest, with an endless queue of passengers. Though the running time was approximately 20 minutes, it stretched close to 30 minutes during rush hours.

Simmons and Boston Colleges became quite hectic which left me very little time to indulge in another of my passions–food. I enjoyed being around food and handling it, so I began working part-time at Star Bucks, located inside the college cafeteria which recharged me thoroughly. The café, Star Bucks, was essentially a place "to see" and "be seen". The smell of freshly-brewed coffee never failed to refresh the exhausted customers, who were mostly students. Chocolate doughnuts, several assortments of muffins, cheese and chocolate croissants, lemon bars, date-and-walnut cakes and jelly rolls comprised the array of bakery items which were accompanied by a variety of frappes and icecream shakes to choose from. It was one of the most exciting jobs I ever had till date!

Leaving home and settling in an unknown city, Boston, which was 3000 miles away from my parents, was difficult to cope with in the beginning. I rented a room in a 300-year-old country-style house which belonged to an American family and was situated on Loveland Road. I found the location convenient and the room quite spacious, which impelled me to book it without looking at any more accommodations. Patty, the home-owner, was Italian by origin. She was a single parent with two daughters, Courtney and Symphony. One of the things I liked best about the place was the lighting. Patty had a fondness for lamps and lit the house with painted antique glass lamps, which added character to the old house. It was soothing and relaxing after a hectic day. The pale green walls reminded me of raw pistachios. The dark mahogany doors, staircase and windows were probably the most expensive items of the house, and ever since her grandma's generation. The antique furniture appropriately suited the house. The dining room had a contemporary touch with a glass-topped dinner table and the modern and well-equipped open kitchen facing it. The crockery was neatly put away inside the glass cabinets. The shelves were stacked with coloured dinner plates, white porcelain bowls and shiny stainless steel cutlery. A few cups and saucers on the kitchen counter had a fine network of cracks, showing signs of aging. The top shelves mostly contained pantry items, loaded with cereals, cookies, and fat-free items for her figure-conscious daughters. There were ketchup, mustard, and tartar sauce jars; tuna fish and cat food for their cat, Rasky; empty mayonnaise bottles which were stacked in one corner of the counter top, were heaped with teabags of endless kinds. The bread basket placed next to the microwave was mostly stuffed with French baguettes, whole-wheat sugar-free bread and soft white sandwich bread. Patty had no salt in her pantry since the bottled spices and herbs already contained salt. Patty and I experimented with food and tried out Indo-American fusion recipes whenever time permitted.

The spiral wooden stairs led to three rooms of which the one on the extreme left was mine. There was a bathroom which was common to all three bedrooms. My room had pink walls, pink drapery and sheets. Too girly, I thought, the first time I saw it. The two windows on adjacent walls of my room let in plenty of sunlight and cross-ventilation. Opposite one of the windows stood an elaborately-carved and polished wooden dresser with a matching wooden-framed mirror.

Another full-length mirror hung on the inside of the wardrobe, in which I hung my daily-wear casuals and jackets. An old antique study table was placed opposite the dresser, facing one of the windows.

The view from the windows included the yard next door, in which the neighbours' German Shepherd snuffled and their toddler splashed in the baby pool. Further beyond, the view stretched to the green patches of land, rooftops of old houses, maple trees tops and sturdy evergreen oaks and hilly pathways. I also got a view of Patty's backyard, which was well-kept with a seasonal herb garden.

In the evenings, the meandering shadows of the tall trees entered my room, while the street lights appeared hazy against the cream-coloured lace curtains. Every time I switched on the lamps, the shadows sped away nowhere.

Besides the rent, I also paid my share of the utility bills. My time with Patty and her daughters was a novel experience. The family accepted me enthusiastically and often inquired about India and our traditional customs. I felt proud talking on behalf of Indians or India as a country. Weekends were the time for grocery shopping, laundry, cooking weekly meals, and other domestic errands. The weekdays slipped by so quickly that on some days even eating required an effort.

I learnt a lot of interesting things that I would not have known had I lived in a dormitory. I learnt that Americans generally brushed their teeth while taking a shower or before going on a date, unlike our morning routine. They also preferred coke or flavoured water to regular water. In Patty's house, breakfast was mostly store-bought from a nearby café consisting of black coffee or latté with a choice of muffins or doughnuts. On weekends their staple brunch consisted of sausage and eggs, "heat-n- eat" pancakes drowning in maple syrup, and bagels or French bread to go with it. On special occasions, or when she felt like cooking, Patty prepared spaghetti with meatballs, their traditional Italian fare which the girls ate with great relish. I sometimes shared a meal with them; I thought Patty cooked well, especially chicken soup and pasta.

Patty and Symphony were friendlier than Courtney, who mostly remained outdoors with her boyfriend, practising soccer. I found it really interesting to see Patty's growing concern that Symphony was not dating boys, unlike her elder daughter Courtney, who went out frequently. Towards the end of my second semester one more girl, who was from Taiwan, rented the adjacent room. Previously the room belonged to one of the girls, but due to Patty's recurrent financial constraints, they decided to rent out the room. Shelby, my new Chinese house mate, was junior to me, completing her under graduation from Berkley College, majoring in music. Now the place was very interesting— an all-women's abode and truly a cultural melting pot! On some weekends, meal-times were a culinary adventure when we enjoyed authentic tastes of China, India and Italy!

Patty had been redoing her basement and bathroom since the time I started living with them. The construction was almost done with the exception of a few fittings, but there was no provision for hot water. The girls seldom used this bathroom because it did not lend itself to their elaborate routine. It was used only in an emergency because of the inconvenience.

Weekday mornings were chaotic with Courtney, Symphony,

Shelby and I competing for the bathroom. Each of us had a routine peculiar to us. On most mornings, Courtney pampered herself with a lavish aromatic bath, after which the bathroom smelled more like a perfume shop. Symphony was the youngest and the slowest! She would occupy the bathroom for so long that it seemed forever, until Patty would bang on the door asking her to hurry up. I normally sneaked in between Symphony's and Shelby's turn. Of course I did not mind that as much as I did with Symphony's habits. Some days, left with no other option, I had to use the basement bathroom and freeze in the shower which did not have any hot water provision. What an experience!

Breakfast, which consisted of a fruit and a sandwich, was mostly on the go as I was required to be at Simmons by 8 am. On weekends it was leisurely, flipping through The New York Times while munching on a bowl of crunchy wheat-cinnamon cereal with soyamilk. Occasionally, I joined Patty's family for brunch. I used to have very long days during the week—I left home early to make it Simmons by 8 am and reached home at night usually after 10. I used to cook for the week during the weekends because of my tight schedule.

It was not the change of place or my lifestyle that converted a fish-eating Bengali girl like me into a vegetarian. I loved vegetarian food even as a child, so there were not too many problems of adjustment with food. I remember Ma would insist that I should taste the fish preparations or other Bengali delicacies that she would prepare. I always enjoyed the vegetarian dishes more than the fish. So, vegetarian food from any cuisine appealed to my palate. I loved the endless variety of salads, soups and different vegetable dishes; but nothing could compare with Ma's cooking. I missed seeing her brisk handling of the ladle as she dropped vegetables into the pan as the hot oil hissed. I sometimes longed for the bite of the mustard and the aroma of spices. Most of all, I missed the way Ma would coax me to try another morsel, because she always felt I did not eat enough.

Sometimes Patty's boyfriend, Daniel, whom she had been seeing for the last thirteen years, ever since her divorce, visited us. Daniel was Jewish, also divorced, and middle-aged as was Patty. He came across as a calm person. He was quite passionate about gardening. He would lovingly cook for Patty; and enjoyed eating too, especially spicy Indian dishes. I think most men have a love affair with food!

He often visited over the weekends from New Hampshire, where he lived from the time Patty had known him. He must have loved visiting a houseful of ladies on weekends! I had once asked Patty if she ever thought of tying the knot with Daniel.

Her reply amazed me when she said, "Sure! I'm only waiting for my girls to get into college because being single I would get grants from the government for their college admission. So you know honey, I can't wait for my girls to leave, after which the real fun would start."

I was awestruck, but managed to smile at her. Often I compared American thinking with ours, and Patty's reply made me think once more! What a commitment— that too for so many years!

****

I Witness a Different World

The best way to help genuinely
is by not being judgmental

Now that you, the reader, know what my growing years were like, which were a contrast to Michele's, it makes it more interesting to know why we very connected so well.

I no longer went through those Monday morning blues once Dr Sparks started counselling me. This week during supervision, besides discussing clients, I thought of expressing my disquiet regarding the influx of new clients as it was beginning to become unmanageable along with the existing ones. Though quite a concern, I chose to discuss it first with other interns to know if they felt similarly.

Dr Sparks became deeply interested to learn about Michele's keenness on initiating conversation regarding our mutual relationship. She indicated that it meant Michele felt quite secure to explore issues that occurred within sessions besides her personal ones. Pausing momentarily she added, "Especially Michele, since I've known her from the time she was with Lisa, isn't the kind to express that openly unless she's thoroughly comfortable." This came to me as a surprise because I presumed maybe she was not that comfortable with me as she had been with Lisa.

"It'll be wise if you begin to lead the sessions, initially, because that will provide directions for her to focus on concrete aspects rather than just exploring weekly updates. Always remember clients' value therapy more when they view it as a place for redefining themselves than simply reiterating their stories," she further advised.

We discussed about Amy and her constant urge to neglect food due to fear of gaining extra pounds. She had mentioned, "I feel like puking if I eat more than two meals a day." This was a big concern for me, since it indicated initial signs of binge eating tendencies. Dr. Sparks insisted on exploring her emotional insecurities, especially relationships. Her insight and guidance always aided my professional growth.

After my supervision, I immersed into my busy client schedule. The entire afternoon flew by with clients, two of whom were new appointments; I felt quite exhausted by the evening. The walk to the train-station was at times tiring although the weather was quite crisp for August.

Finally it was Friday— the weekend! I got time off on Fridays since I had no classes scheduled at Boston College. On some days I visited the library to catch up with pending reference or research work, on other days I preferred relaxing to go out with friends for dinner, or spend time watching F.R.I.E.N.D.S with Patty and the gang of girls.

At the Counselling Centre, however, Friday mornings were cramped with group supervision, intern meetings and other staff meetings for the forthcoming week. Mornings flew by almost in the blink of eye, especially after the meetings and back-to-back sessions, Michele being the last one. It was from the fourth session that Michele unlocked her pain and the fears she had been carrying since for quite some time. She was scheduled for an early session that Friday.

1 August, 2003

Session: 4

Michele arrived precisely on time, at 2 pm, wearing her infectious smile. She seemed relaxed and greeted me, "I was longing to see you. Ever since I've started exploring my past, weird thoughts have been coming to my mind."

"Are those thoughts pertaining to you?," I asked. She did not reply and shifted her gaze to the floor rug. Tears rolled down her cheeks as she started crying. I waited for a couple of minutes before asking her the cause for her sadness.

She complained, "Mom accused me last night on the phone and passed sarcastic comments for not performing well academically. Mom called to inquire about my grades. As long as I have been in Simmons, never has she called to inquire if I adjusted well in Boston, or where I was living. All she's concerned about is my academic result."

"How often does she call?"

Michele declared, "Thank goodness she does not call often! Whenever she does, it always ends with sarcasm."

On my probing she elaborated, "Mom once laughed with disbelief when I informed her about my project being selected as the best in class. Instead of feeling proud of me or happy for me, she said that I must have copied the idea from somewhere because my work would not have got that much recognition."

I was quite surprised to hear those comments and inquired, "Is there anything specific that she dislikes about you? How long has this been going on?"

"She dislikes me as a person. Gosh! I don't remember how long, but it has been this way ever since I recall."

She wiped her tears and admitted feeling lighter discussing her concern aloud. After lingering some more on the matter, Michele began talking on an entirely different topic.

"Actually there is something else I wanted to share with you," she announced looking unsure, "Jane, who's my roommate and my classmate as well, now lives with me. We decided to move in together in an apartment a couple of weeks ago, instead of staying in the dorm. We share the rent; Jane works part-time after classes and I arrange mine through on-campus assistantships."

I wondered what triggered Michele to discuss Jane. However, I remained open to all her thoughts. "Actually, we both are going around as partners. I was attracted towards her since I met her in class and my interest escalated knowing that she was a lesbian too. We've been dating ever since. We share wonderful emotional and sexual intimacy. But then…sometimes I feel guilty dating a woman and I don't know if I can date men ever again!"

"I think maybe you are still exploring and undecided if Jane is the right person for you. Also being attracted towards both sexes, being bisexual, that is, is quite likely to happen among many persons of your age. This is more of an exploratory phase as you begin experimenting through new relationships. However, I don't see any reason to feel guilty about it since this is quite natural. It isn't possible to convert sexual orientations wishfully; I'm sure you will agree on that!"

Michele listened to my little speech attentively, and stated, "Maybe you are right. This is a sort of self-discovery! I did feel attracted to guys initially, as I had mentioned earlier; but after being with Jane, I feel this is what I have always wanted. But I feel bad thinking about my parents and how they would react after knowing that I am a lesbian or may be bisexual. I often feel embarrassed displaying my affection to Jane in public, though she doesn't. Sometimes I think of breaking up with her and to date men to see if it works; but then I don't want to lose her either. It's a dilemma I haven't been able to share with anyone."

I questioned if she felt embarrassed accepting herself as a lesbian. Michele agreed that she did feel ashamed because of the social pressures and especially feared the reactions of her family. "The deeper I indulge in such thoughts the more I get confused. I'm still not comfortable to refer myself as a lesbian. Also, Jane is the first person with whom I want to continue long-term unlike the previous men I dated. It is ….it is like…like ….I wish I could explain."

I helped her focus, "Like a maze, where you walk without knowing where or what point you may reach."

"Precisely," she added.

"Is it the fear of your mother that makes you uncomfortable identifying yourself as a lesbian?," I inquired.

"I was never too close to Mom so I don't expect her to love me anyway! However, I fear being subjected to her anger and sarcasm. In fact, she might despise me even more, discovering my relationship with another woman. I will always remain the 'bad girl' and, of course, Emily-the 'good girl' of the family."

Michele mumbled the words, "bad girl" several times while gazing at the floor rug until I spoke.

"I am sorry to know about your relationship with your mother, but what makes you think of yourself as a bad girl?"

Michele continued, "I decided to live away from home only to be away from Mom. She always picked on me. Everything I did, said, planned or liked, was wrong but whatever Emily did, thought, or said was appreciated and accepted. The constant comparison has haunted me throughout my childhood. I started losing confidence, being trapped within this vicious negativity. When I got admission in Simmons, Mom mocked me that Emily would go to a better reputed college than mine. I know my sister is prettier and academically stronger, but is it all that relationships are made of or based on? My artwork always remained unnoticed. My 'A' grades in English remained next to unimportant, my language skills and vocabulary were always disregarded. She always pointed out the flaws, drawing unnecessary negative conclusions about my behaviour. My childhood experiences are my worst memories and I have started believing, "I am a bad girl."

"Sorry for what you went through. Have you ever spoken to your mother about your feelings and asked her why she behaves this way with you?," I asked empathetically.

She shook her head in denial.

Michele continued, "I am tired of Mom. During childhood, the more I strove to connect with her, the worse it became so now I've left hope. I feel relationships are mean, isolations are peaceful comparatively!"

Reiterating her thoughts I said, "You seem to be hurt and neglected by your mother. It must be frustrating too!"

"Totally frustrating and I have felt this way since long. Sometimes I wish I could replace my Mom, like clothes!" she exclaimed.

I thought that was quite a strong statement but due to time constraints I had to wrap up the topic. "Today you touched on several aspects from your past. We would work through them and see how it goes. It is not easy to recollect unpleasant moments and walk out erasing all of those thoughts instantly. I hope you will be able to manage and keep your calm after the session." "Thanks for your concern, I got a bit carried away thinking of my Mom, but I'll be just fine," she reassured me.

After the session ended, I felt as if layers of grey-black clouds of words hovered over my head. The intensity of pain she expressed throughout the session from her childhood sorrows to her present love-life confusions, almost overwhelmed me. Tears, shame, self-blame, and love all were tapped in one session. I wrote the following about the session:

Process Notes

Session: 4

This week Michele unlocked her apprehensions and wept all through as she spoke about her Mom. She fears that her sexual identity might exclude her completely from her family. I was a bit confused that she still thought about dating men in spite of being with Jane. Michele felt somewhat embarrassed disclosing this, but was glad that she did.

I noticed her tearful, sad eyes today.

It seemed Michele is unknowingly internalizing her mother's thoughts and, therefore, feeling guilty for making choices according to her heart's desire. This has started impacting her self-esteem as well.

I began winding up after finishing the notes on Michele. While at the Fenway stop, my mind raced in different directions with myriad thoughts, questions and analyses. Though I wanted to visit the library to finish previous week's pending work, the session had consumed all my energy. Stress due to work had weakened my appetite, so I decided to pick up only a sandwich for dinner on my way back home. I did not do much after my return besides enjoying my store-bought sandwich and conversing on the phone. I went to bed soon after as I wanted to be rested the next morning. I was awakened past midnight by the sound of giggles and familiar voices; it was probably Patty and her daughters. Disinterested, I went back to sleep again.

The weekend was busy as usual and I did not have much spare time. I looked forward most to Saturday evenings, because it was the only time I got for socializing. Boston being the cultural hub of plays and dramas, my two close friends, Amanda and Teri, and I occasionally frequented the theatres after having lunch at one of our favourite Thai restaurants. After all that fun, Sunday remained generally the day to prepare for the week ahead.

****

Monday mornings started with group meetings and individual supervision. These meetings were quite handy to resolve any doubts pertaining to clients. During supervision I openly expressed my slight hesitation about dealing with a lesbian client for the first time. Initially, I felt awkward sitting with her or imagining her with another woman, though I approved of it as her personal choice. As I attended to her childhood experiences and her desire for finding true compassion along with her fear of being identified as a lesbian, I became more attached to her issues professionally. I am glad that in spite of belonging to a culture where homosexuality is a thing of taboo, I could genuinely empathize with Michele. My private counselling sessions with her added towards this openness largely.

During supervision I realized that she was no different than I or any other person merely because of her sexual orientation and as a counsellor I needed to simply accept and support her thoughts.

In course of the session, Dr Sparks complimented me which felt great! She said, "It's true that sexual orientation, because it is so personal, demands a comfort zone before one can disclose it to others. I would feel honoured, if I were you, to be trusted within such short number of sessions by a client."

I was gratified to hear that; and went on to discuss my next clients stationed in line were Rupa, Beth and Amy and their respective dilemmas.

Dr Sparks elaborated, "The best way is to let the client head the sessions or decide what they want to explore. Clients are quite directive and will often tell you, either explicitly or subtly, about what they expect. Follow your clients by listening to them closely, verbally as well as non-verbally. Also, it might help if you imagined yourself in that situation and how you might have reacted."

I had learnt in theory that counselling is a two-way process where both the client and the counsellor grow and discover themselves in yet another new dimension, which was becoming true for me in the real sense.

Later, I introspected further, while travelling back to Boston College, and found myself adding new thoughts as a result of her suggestions. With time, I knew my clients were not just some unknown individuals who came to me with their problems, they had become more than that for me. Maybe it was not professional, but I felt bad when things went wrong in their lives. Some clients even influenced me on a personal level such as Michele made me anxious at times, and while sitting with Rupa I often felt irritated. However, these were my internalized feelings that I seldom displayed during sessions.

Another habit of mine, with which I struggled often, was an urge to state my opinions before the client could do so. Being talkative by nature, it was challenging for me to talk less and listen more efficiently as a counsellor. However, I noticed that when I remained silent and allowed the clients to take over the sessions were more insightful. Therapy actually works wonders when most of the talking, feedback, and insight come from the clients; instead of counsellor probing with suggestions and new ideas. Letting the clients explore unhindered lends them a chance to take risks and experiment with their thoughts openly. It is interesting that even though counsellors possess more command within the professional parameters, it is the client who ultimately makes the process successful or not with their final word.

In the course of time, I began applying my theoretical knowledge and expertise from Boston College into practical use in sessions.

Previously, I had engaged in client-counsellor role-plays with pseudo-issues, but that was nothing compared to the actual experience. I was able to nurture a trustworthy bond with my clients, who confided in me their darkest secrets, fears and deep-rooted concerns, so much so that sometimes I felt I was responsible for their well-being. As their lives unfolded before me through the sessions, they made me aware of many life situations that I would not have known otherwise. It was amazing, at times, to experience different worlds, hitherto unknown, through clients' narratives. This was not just about counselling, but was also a part of my own learning process.

****

Counselling Myself

Self-criticism is our best friend
in the process of growing

My Master's programme was so demanding that even when I was home, I was typing papers; and allowed lesser and lesser opportunities to spend time socializing. Life was a whirlwind, with the increasing load of work with each succeeding semester.

In between academics, I found interest in dealing with clients. Their issues and concerns awakened me to the realities of life even more. I had never encountered anorexic women before and to actually sit with one over repeated sessions was itself a learning process. Rupa, with whom I had so much common being the fact we both were Indians, but her skepticism always kept me at a distance from her. It is rather discomforting when I thought Indians were probably my toughest clients.

I was required to do a research project on the origin and formation of family in the family therapy class. Some of the findings were intriguing, such as: origins of a family began with monkeys and chimpanzees. One of my assignments in family therapy was analyzing our own family histories, the prejudices, cultural background and other aspects. Initially, my shyness and vulnerability to disclose personal issues impeded my ability to analyse. In the beginning it was tough to disclose facts because it caused discomfort to me. I was reluctant to criticise or bring to light the negative points of my family, but this was temporary and I accepted it as a part of the learning process.

My clients indirectly had tutored me with the right amount of confidence needed to expressive sensitive private concerns, although my situation was different from theirs. Over the course of writing instead of judging the wrongs and rights I began to perceive the context under which those actions occurred and becoming more accepting of them.

In the course of discussing details about my family, the power dynamics, negotiations, openness to communication and diplomacy, I became aware of insights that I had not been aware of so far.

While with clients or discussing the family dynamics of my fellow-students, I realized how fortunate I was, after hearing accounts of broken families, foster-care upbringing and other distorted relational problems. In class, many of my classmates shared their experiences of parental discord or divorce or memories of growing up in foster homes, a lot of it being quite painful to share. I thought Indians had strong family bonds, by and large, where the children had a far more sheltered life. By the time I finished the final draft of the paper, I felt quite good about myself that I had freed myself from many constraints to write about my family without concealing any facts. I became cognizant and perceived situations with transparency instead of looking through these with tinted glasses which are provided to us by society.

With subsequent courses such as Multicultural Issues, Counselling Women, Issues in Life Span, Drug and Alcohol Abuse, and LGBT (Lesbian, Gay, Bisexual, Transgender) Issues, I candidly began to acknowledge and accept the changes that one goes through in life. I inferred that weaknesses or shortcomings did not make an individual good or bad, unless they presented themselves so. The process sensitized me towards others, and relationship issues in general, which wasn't the case earlier. I realized that people are more or less similar the world over, though their language, appearance, and lifestyle are varied. All emotions in their true sense are worthy of acceptance, be it crying to express sorrow or shouting when angry.

None of these emotions are bad because they help depict our underlying feelings. The problem occurs when we misinterpret our emotions and label it as negative or suppress it. Anger is as important an emotion as love is; only expressed differently. Trouble starts when a single emotion dominates an individual's personality such as too much love can lead to overprotection or curb the other person's personal space.

Besides professional competence, self-counselling facilitated a more rational understanding of personal relationship. It permitted me to accept others with greater flexibility and transparency. Counselling honed my skill to listen and comprehend circumstances from the other person's perspective without losing my own individuality.

Those who are not familiar with counselling, here is a brief insight into how it actually works. This is a process of continuous interaction between two individuals as they connect, communicate and contemplate. It aims at intrinsically valuing individuals for the persons they are, irrespective of their right or wrong actions, feelings or experiences. The counsellor acts as a facilitator to expedite and to clients think more clearly. It is a space where there are no façades, judgments, opinions or advice. As counselling progresses, the clients learn to self-evaluate their own actions according to the given situation. The ultimate goal is to help clients take decisions on their own in such a way that it does not interfere with their identity, confidence and self-esteem. This unconditional sharing experience with the counsellor, where the client is not judged sets it apart from discussing the same with a friend or family member, thus endorsing trust within the counsellor-client relationship. All information shared is kept confidential.

In practice, though, I witnessed ample diverse connotations of this process. Ideally, empathetic behaviour and unconditional acceptance works wonders, but sometimes clients have a problem trusting their counsellor, to the extent that they cross-question prior to disclosing any information. In such cases, establishment of rapport itself takes couple of sessions. Abrupt terminations are common in case clients are not dedicated or persistent. It is not unusual for new counsellors to blame themselves or have their confidence shaken on account of such terminations. In they face of such occurrences exploring such concerns and misconceptions with a supervisor becomes necessary to resolve such feelings.

****

Another aspect that added significantly to my professional growth was seeking counselling for myself. It was necessary, at that time, to manage my own emotions and the daily wear-and-tear by clients. I visited the counsellor at Boston College though it did not work out well. Soon I terminated my sessions with him. I started seeing Dr Sparks, my supervisor, for personal counselling sessions. In addition to being an incredible supervisor, I found her to be an excellent therapist. We connected instinctively, maybe because I was already acquainted with her during supervision.

There were doubts and unknown fears, some professional, most were personal, which we explored. I became more transparent and accepted imperfection as an integral part of myself, and did not feel embarrassed to discuss them explicitly. I was learning to know myself with a new insight. Nothing had been this interesting and exciting than discovering my own behavioural patterns and the reasons behind such patterns.

We all love to display our good qualities and strengths, but what happens to our darker side? Yes, we do have one and it does not change overnight, which means most of us either hide or ignore it. Dr Sparks facilitated me to recognize my negative points as much as my positive qualities as an integral part of myself. I further appreciated that there was no need to present myself perfectly to others by hiding my shortcomings. It is true that our continuous struggle to be faultless to "others" and to "self" often steals our true nature. Moreover, concepts like perfection and self-esteem are too elusive and they vary from person to person. Positives of one can be negatives of another person. She explained, "You need to be aware of your irrational behaviour in order to improve. Self-acceptance is the key to confidence and high self-esteem."

There were times when I cried during sessions and it was a relief to do so. I acknowledged missing my family and the challenge of living alone in a completely unknown city. Dr Sparks supported and reminded me by pointing out the positive aspects of living alone such as the independence and growth that would not have been possible without accepting this challenge. She seldom spoke during sessions and the little that she did was towards the end while sharing her thoughts. My counselling sessions truly enlightened me.

I cherished every moment of experiencing the other side, that is, as a client, and believed that in order to understand their clients better, counsellors should consider counselling themselves as a part of their training. For instance, my counsellor at Boston College mostly jotted all the factual information I presented, with very little eye contact, which I found quite distracting. After being aware of such an occurrence, I tried not to repeat the same mistake by keeping my written notes to a minimum. Though such details might seem trivial but they go a long way in forming a rapport with the clients.

I shared my euphoria with Dr Sparks, on seeing my clients come back for sessions consistently. Much of it was the excitement of actually counselling clients and the newness of the process. Reiterating my childhood and growing experiences during self-counselling I felt as if I was truly reliving those moments again.

I remember my childhood to be a treasure-chest of positive memories. I am extremely fortunate to have been brought up within a contemporary open-minded family. In spite of being the only child I was not pampered but was somewhat overprotected to be the centre of attention at all times. I wondered how different my childhood would have been with siblings though I never regretted their absence since my extended family and friends compensated for that loneliness.

Ma became my best friend as I grew older. Generally it is seen daughters to be more attached with their fathers than their mothers, but my case was different. Throughout my growing years I knew her to be one of the most balanced and optimistic persons who always considered the positive side of life. Our communication was unlike that of parent and child and more like friends. Ma has always been beside me with her unstinting support, encouragement and advice, helping me with every decision of mine–even clothing! I admire her melodious voice and her incredible memory which enables her to remember dates and events with accuracy despite passing years.

With my Baba the equation changes, we are quite unlike each other in temperament, though I resemble him, He is rational, systematic and more practical than I. Despite our difference in our approach, there has been no problem of communication. I can always speak my heart out and know that he would understand. He never imposed his opinion on me but listened to my arguments with patience, which brought us closer over the years. He is very affectionate and absolutely wonderful listener, which works well for me and Ma since we love to talk! He is my critic for all the new culinary recipes I try, my mentor in professional decision-making, and the person who loves me the most and undoubtedly worries the maximum. Baba has always been extra cautious about matters pertaining to me, may be because I am the only child. The more I think the more I realize and accept that it is a blessing to be born to any parents.

School, my second home, taught me to multi-task and become

connected to the world of knowledge. It was wonderful to share lunch-boxes during break-time, to exchange jokes and laugh during classes and many countless experiences. Besides, I learnt to eat breakfast quickly in the morning and not dawdle. I was more comfortable being a follower than a leader. As long as I worked in groups jointly on projects and symposiums it was fun, but felt hesitant when it came to performing alone. Simply standing up and reading in front of the class was an ordeal for me.

I remember how much I dreaded the literature classes when new chapters were introduced. Mrs Mukherji, our English teacher, would call out names and ask them to read the chapter aloud to the class. I remember my hands would turn sweaty during my turn and my mouth would go dry when it was my turn to read. Inevitably I would mispronounce certain words out of sheer self-consciousness. But the real embarrassment would come when Mrs Mukherji would correct me and there would be a titter of giggles from some students at the back. "Be a little louder" was a constant refrain that accompanied my readings. Once I was done with my turn it was such a relief as if I had not gagged while swallowing bitter medicine. These incidents of junior classes now seem so inconsequential but may have been the reason why initially conducting sessions alone with clients made me feel anxious at times.

In college, however, I became more interactive and took an active part in solo discussions as well. All my childhood vulnerabilities, performance, anxieties, shyness faded as I began specializing in my choice of subjects and courses. Popularity among friends, appreciation and recognition from family and mentors instilled confidence in me. Majoring in Psychology from Jesus and Mary College in Delhi not only furthered my pursuit to do Master's in the subject, but also etched the finest memories to last a lifetime. Besides academics, the canteen gossip, endless servings of *bhelpuris, sevpuris, keema samosas*, library visits, bunking classes to watch movies at Chanakya, the theatre situated closest to college, sneaking out of tiring practical classes, added to the timeless memories.

I began embarking on my journey of exploration of life with people from different walks of life. My scope of knowledge in Psychology, especially counselling, widened limitlessly with the courses offered in Boston College. Interestingly, I never felt conscious about my pronunciation or speaking ability in Boston College, unlike as I did back in school, although my class had a large number of students whose first language was English. Life was beginning to take shape like a lump of clay spinning on the potter's wheel.

****

I Am Inspired to Explore

Ignorance is worse than fear; let my spirits
rise free beyond the obvious, towards enlightenment

Michele became my inspiration to discover and educate myself about the gay/lesbian community. My knowledge in this regard was sketchy until then. Simultaneously, I thought about the scope of studying homosexuality in India, which would not have been the same as it is not discussed openly in Indian society. The aspect of homosexuality is not new in India. There are several examples of it depicted in Indian mythology The royal harems during the middle ages were guarded by eunuchs or, at times, transgenders. Contemporary poetry abounds with references to homosexual love. Social anthropologists are of the opinion that it was the Victorian ethos and attitude which changed the liberal thinking. As a result our society tries to avoid explicit discussions on such issues and condemns such behaviour in both covert and overt ways.

In the United States, this was certainly not the case and I got ample opportunities to augment my knowledge. I was also fortunate at the time to sign up for a course at Boston College-Counselling

Gay/Lesbian Community. This further widened my understanding of several sensitive issues that they face and interventions to deal with such issues. It educated me about low self-esteem, negative thinking, fear and the inferiority complex, which the community often faces. The learning programme was truly beneficial not only for working with clients who were dealing with such issues, but also to expand my own horizon of awareness. The process eliminated preconceived notions and myths such as homosexuality is due to stress and less than ideal parenting, or bottled up frustrations and that bisexuality is a transitional phase between heterosexuality and homosexuality. I was unaware, till then, due to my limited knowledge and experience, that bisexuals are as prevalent a community as gay and lesbians. Confidence, clarity, and compassion were the three C's I learnt through this journey.

Interestingly, most of the participants attending the course supported the cause of the LGBT community. However, a few, though they were counsellors themselves, were not inclined to be supportive; perhaps because of their faith, which was Catholicism. During my interaction with those people, I thought of Michele's mother, who was also Catholic. The course gave me an impetus to deal with clients more effectively in this area. I wrote down my thoughts in my personal dairy which I maintained during the course, which I want to share here:

Gay, lesbian, bisexual or heterosexual are all tags we allot to ourselves to become aware of our sexual preferences. I put forth that sexual orientation is a capacity to be rather than a restriction. It means we are gifted to unconditionally love a person to fulfil our own emotional, spiritual, social and sexual desires. In this context, it is of less significance whether the loved one is of the same sex or not. A recurrent or continued fondness for the same, referred as homosexuality, is just another choice one makes, much like choosing between a love and an arranged marriage. A woman may find other women more physically attractive than men but in no way should that impede her personality development or the right to live with respect. Ultimately it comes down to personal choices, of what one feels comfortable with and asserting it desirably. A homosexual or heterosexual identity must not interfere or hinder with the intellectual and emotional enhancement of individuals. It is simply another aspect of identity of a person as are his/her religion, sex, language or nationality.

I also became responsive to the common mistakes we often commit unknowingly that might show insensitivity towards others. For instance, in job application forms, sex has only two categories–male and female; second, the assumption that people will always have partners of the opposite sex are examples of heterosexist behaviour. Especially in India, I feel, sexual orientation is taken for granted, thereby failing to recognize other possibilities. Mockery and ridiculing comments seem to have become an inherent part in the lives of gays/lesbians. Parents mostly feel embarrassed to accept their children as homosexuals; they would rather suppress or disregard such emotions as baseless or immoral.

It is not surprising when such reactions force them to conceal their real identities and live a life of pretence, which leads to loss of confidence and the feeling of self-loathing. Isolation from friends and family, increased use of alcohol consumption, depression, low self-esteem and suicidal attempts become common symptoms among the community. Counselling, in this case, acts as a safe space for displaying such thoughts explicitly in the absence of societal fear or any sort of criticism. The therapist needs to assist and support the client by showing unconditional empathy.

"Coming out" is a term referred to an individual's effort to openly declare his/her homosexuality to their family, friends, and other acquaintances. This is one of the most challenging phases one encounters because it has the potential to break or make relationships, and can be quite taxing on their mental health as well. Counselling addresses these sensitive issues, fears, and explores ways to deal with the "coming out" process. Support and a non-judgmental attitude of the counsellor helps to bring back the client's lost confidence, positive self-esteem and feelings of being worthy as an individual. To widen my scope further, I indulged in reading books related to such issues, discovering the obvious and not so obvious facts, and the societal dos and don'ts in this context.

A sense of fulfilment surged through me when I found myself behaving at ease and with compassion with my homosexual clients. Despite acquiring quite some familiarity on the possible issues, reality often displayed intricate complications with unique circumstances for each of the clients whom I counselled.

My course at Boston College refined my theoretical knowledge and other aspects, such as, rigidity towards those having same-sex partners, negative attitude of family members, who try to change the person's sexual orientation with treatments or medicines, and other behavioural disorders. I was fortunate to attend a couple of workshops, one of them especially designed for gays/lesbians to help them deal with stereotypical remarks and comments from the not so well-informed section of straight population. I wished such workshops were arranged in India as they were an excellent way to bring about awareness and potential changes among people. This was not an easy process for me as well; it took time and effort to instil such awareness within me. Initially, because I was ill-informed on such matters I could not relate well to the feelings and emotions of homosexual clients.

Putting myself in my client's shoes I could not imagine how it would feel romancing with another woman. Being straight, I always had to remind myself to listen carefully to the romantic feelings of my lesbian clients. Similar to any relationship, they also underwent similar concerns like giving spaces to each other or making compromises. However, social humiliation and the fear of being judged were added constraints among same-sex couples.

****

I was beginning to feel enlightened by the knowledge I had accumulated through all these interventions and interactions with the community. At Simmons, I decided to arrange a forum for an open-house discussion on "Societal Dissonance towards Gays/lesbians". The purpose of this was to generate awareness among the youth and to get their feedback on such issues. The overwhelming response from the students and staff accelerated the success of the forum. I was surprised when a couple of students openly confessed their stereotypical outlook and viewed same-sex couples with reservations. Some allegedly put forth that heterosexuality is only feasible and lawful way to relationships. However, promoters defended it by holding sexual orientation to be a personal choice. Guest speakers spoke on the same to support flexibility and approachable communication channels within peer groups and families of gays and lesbians. I felt gratified to promote awareness among students. The forum was not aimed to change views overnight; it was only an attempt to sow the seeds of awareness.

Since my latest preoccupation was the welfare of lesbian community, Michele continually lingered at the back of my mind all week long. I wondered if she had attended the open house and I was curious to get her feedback.

"Relationships are mean, isolations are peaceful", Michele's words from the previous session, kept me wondering if counselling could undo such fears. My eyes moistened slightly as I thought of her and felt like hugging her to let her know that this was just a phase and it would pass. By now, I knew I had a special place for Michele, though it was a little difficult to accept this client initially. My eagerness to see her this week escalated as Friday approached.

Although my schedule was crammed with classes, clients and also such outdoor activities at Simmons, I did not feel as exhausted and got more work done than usual! I was thoroughly engulfed with my course work and clients. My effort to educate myself did not go in vain as it profusely paid off when dealing with clients undergoing sexual identity crises. Besides gaining a humungous amount of knowledge, the experience was like diving into a pool and discovering a river.

****

Heartbreak

Listening becomes a treasure when
our heart listens between the lines

The rest of the week flew and soon it was Thursday night; I was lulled to sleep with the soft sounds of the night coming through the window. I woke up before the alarm rang and leapt out of bed. I looked out of the window and saw the sky turn pink and gold as the sun glowed softly and as fresh as if it was the first dawn ever. It was Friday, and the weekend was around the corner. I quickly took a shower, had breakfast of a bowl of cereal and rushed out towards the train-stop, "The Reservoir."

It was only a month since internship had begun at Simmons and we all could already feel the stress piling up. Our director, Dr Jonathan, addressed some housekeeping and ethical issues that needed to be checked with all the interns. Safety of suicidal clients and severely-depressed ones were given special attention during the meeting. My usual array of clients continued thereafter and I followed their lives as keenly as I always did. I had my second last session with Beth. It was my fourth session with her. She seemed quite depressed mostly and her weekly accounts mostly consisted of her deep longing for her family and her lover back in Ireland. Interestingly, she never shed tears. With Beth I often felt she felt tried hard to control her emotions. Once she reported, "If I am able to restrict my sadness, I feel less like a loser." Sessions with her were like breaking a chunk of ice. She challenged me with every escalating session.

Michele was my last client for the day following Beth.

8 August, 2003

Session: 5

Michele, as always, was on time for her fifth session. She greeted me enthusiastically and I instantly felt that she was better and happier than the previous week.

She began after settling down in the chair, "I attended the talk show that you had arranged and thought it was totally cool–such an eye-opener for the ignorant lots!"

I noticed her smile broadly.

She continued, "Yes, this is important but not everything can be discussed openly. You know what I mean."

When I asked her to clarify on what she meant specifically she explained it with her own life. "For instance, I can share my experiences only with those whom I feel would understand me, not with everyone I know."

"Do you feel you have to be perfect to share your life with others?," I asked her. Michele hesitantly replied, "No…not exactly, I don't know. Yes, maybe! Since I have never had a perfect life, I really can't talk about it."

"What is a perfect life for you?,"

Michele thought for a while before she spoke, "Uh! I like that question…what is perfect life? Well, for me I would think if my parents accept me the way I am without criticism and my results improve, I'd be quite happy as of now. However, in the future I'd like to be with my ideal partner, a beautiful house, a secure job and the list goes on and on."

"Okay, so you feel this would take away all your problems in life and make you more confident to share your life experiences with others?," I questioned.

She was silent for a while. Shrugging her shoulders, Michele clarified her statement, "No, I don't think a problem-free life is possible but I wish it were so."

"It's your own attitude and optimistic thoughts that makes life smooth. Each one of us goes through hurdles; it's the way we deal with it, which deems us a winner or a loser."

She nodded understandinglyat my words.

Then pausing momentarily Michele continued, "I wanted to discuss about Jane actually. You remember her right, my partner and roommate?"

"Of course I do," I urged.

"You know I and Jane are romantically involved since the last three-four months now. Things were moving fine and I really felt good about us being together. Jane is the assertive one, often indulging in PDA though I feel a bit awkward at times, like she doesn't mind kissing me in a store."

I added, "Probably that's her way of loving you and showing

affection. Also, she doesn't mind letting the world know about her identity, which you seem to be struggling with at the moment."

Michele agreed, "Yes! Sometimes I wonder if she does it to grab attention of others especially the other girls around. You know she's the kind of person who could make friends with just about anyone; she is very outgoing and extremely confident."

I asked her, "Does that work well with you? Is that a good thing?"

"Yes and no, actually", Michele replied thoughtfully, "Her confidence and vision of the future of our relationship boosts my will-power, while her extroverted and demonstrative behaviour sometimes causes me apprehension and last Sunday's incident really shook me."

"I was supposed to go home last weekend so I came early for the session as well. We hugged and kissed before I left; it was the first time we would be away from each other. I promised to call every night. I reached the airport well before time to avoid the evening traffic. At the check-in counter there was a crowd which was noisy. I managed to reach the counter and found that my flight was cancelled due to bad weather conditions. I was slightly disappointed because the next flight to Ohio was early morning next day. I had not visited home for long and Emily had insisted to get together over the weekend, but all my efforts went in vain. I decided to head back and, of course, surprise Jane. I didn't bother to call because we have duplicate keys and I'm glad I didn't call."

Michele had made reasonable eye contact with me until then, but eventually she started gazing at the rug. Sensing that something had upset her more than just a cancelled flight, I remarked, "I think something affected you deeply."

"Yes it did and it still hurts!" she exclaimed, "Our apartment door was unlocked, and I walked in, wanting to surprise Jane. Instead, I found Jane making love with another woman. They were wrapped in each other's arms, with Jane passionately kissing her naked back. I was stunned and felt disgusted. I shouted and rushed outside into the living room. I could not stand the sight of their intimacy. Gosh! I couldn't believe my eyes!"

Michele's face went red as she expressed her rage. She burst into tears, "She cheated me. I had trusted Jane the most ever since we met and now everything's over."

"Michele, did you talk to Jane, as to why she did it? It must be really hard being betrayed by the one you deeply love."

"I hadn't seen Jane so nervous before. She could hardly speak—I was so shattered–I was shrieking and shouting with the pain and shock. I had seen Dory, Jane's new love, a couple of times in the cafeteria, but never really interacted. I thought her to be a docile person, but certainly not after this incident!"

Continuing on the same note she continued, "Jane began shedding crocodile tears after Dory left. Generally, I could not bear to see Jane crying, but her actions had flushed out all my sympathy. I slammed the door and dashed out to breathe some fresh air and speculated repeatedly if Jane did it under some compulsion. I wanted to believe that I was hallucinating, all this was a joke and that she still loved me, but I was wrong. I could not justify her behaviour."

Glancing at her pale face I nodded.

"Later that night, Jane apologized and confessed about Dory's unexpected visit that led to such an impulsive act. She admitted being sexually aroused by Dory's voluptuous figure and had lost control. Dory already had a boyfriend, but did not mind experimenting either! I feel sorry for her boyfriend. It seems the world is full of greedy sexually-charged animals!" Michele exclaimed angrily this time.

I saw disgust, hurt, anger and hatred in her expression; she needed to confront her feelings and get past them; and that is what I let her do.

"It isn't easy to set aside such experiences so quickly," I added.

"I feel lonely, cut loose, as if belonging nowhere."

"I don't intend to hurt you; but would you have preferred to have been ignorant about this truth?"

She caught my words instantly, "I know it's good that I came to know about it, but still, it hurts."

"It will hurt and that is quite natural. Well, now you know how those persons might have felt, whom you left because of another person or when you fell out of love with them."

After a brief pause, Michele wiped her tears and her nose with the stack of tissues placed on the corner table, and stated, "I agree with what you said. Perhaps it wasn't right what I did with Darren and the rest of them. But at least I was honest about my feelings and insisted on breaking up because I didn't want to betray them, unlike Jane who was actually two-timing."

She creased her brows and declared with conviction, "I'm thinking of moving out soon and rent a cheaper place all by myself since there aren't any vacancies in the dorm. The sooner the better!

It's awkward to live with Jane now since we aren't talking any more. Rather, I try to avoid her more."

Although living with Jane was getting harder by the day for her, I expressed my concern for her safety as she was planning to move out and live alone. Michele thanked me and said, "At least someone cares."

"It was good to vent my emotions. I feel lighter after talking to you, also because I hadn't shared this with anyone yet," she ended.

Time slipped away like sand in an hour-glass. After Michele left, I stretched myself gingerly. My lower back was hurting; it felt stiff from sitting in one position all day long glued to the "listening chair."

On my way back, I walked through the premises of Simmons College towards the train-stop. The evening sun shone on the evergreen pine trees which were lined along Fenway Avenue. It was a pleasantly cool evening, unlike Delhi in August. Rows of runners ran past me, dressed in multicoloured shorts and tees. I felt happy simply watching their energy; it almost took away all my fatigue.

After I reached home, I did some stretching exercises. It felt great straightening my spine after all the day's work. I slipped a padded cushion for support behind my back and rested for a while before having a light dinner. I was too tired that night and decided to fill in my notes the following morning.

It was fresh and crisp outside when I woke up. I got out of bed and slipped on my black-and white-spotted chappals, which I had got from India and walked to the window. The view was quiet, nothing like the mornings in India. No noise of buses and auto-rickshaws honking. The foliage looked fresh and dewy, with the vibrant yellow flowers and lush green grass. I changed into my walking shoes, track-pants and sweat-shirt and stepped out for a quick stroll. I was glad I did it! It was breathtakingly beautiful outside. The pathways were wet as it had rained the previous night, the leaves and flowers still had droplets on them. Nature had been very generous with her bounty in the case of Boston. However, I could not linger for long as pending work beckoned. I spent my afternoon finishing my work which also included the process notes for Michele. This is what I jotted down for her:

Process notes: 5

Michele felt depressed and betrayed for all the love and trust she had showered on her girlfriend. Her faith in relationships seems to have been shaken once again after reviving from issues with her mother.

While listening I was also paying attention to all her non-verbal cues. Michele clutched her hands tightly, as if trying to gain courage to speak up. I felt extremely sorry for her and felt her pain but there wasn't much to say.

I visualized the scene, as she spoke, Michele crying, Jane and Dory too embarrassed to confess and so forth. I was reminded of the famous saying— a mirror once cracked never becomes the same again. There was a positive note; during our conversation, she realized that it was good she became aware of Jane's true nature within a couple of months of their relationship.

****

One good thing was I got to attend an American wedding over the weekend. It was wholly a new experience for me. I had never been to a Catholic wedding in a church before. My friend, who was the bride, looked stunning in her white lace gown. The men were equally attractive in their black Tuxedos. I constantly kept comparing our Indian wedding routine sporadically throughout the ceremony. As grand as the wedding was, personally I preferred a gorgeous Indian wedding.

The new week marked a milestone in my growth as a counsellor. Over the week things paced pretty fast. Besides all other stuff, I hoped Michele had found a suitable apartment for herself; and was waiting to see her eagerly in session.

15 August, 2003

Session: 6

Michele greeted me as she walked in on her scheduled time. I inquired on her latest happenings.

"Just about okay, I guess!" she answered, "My quest for a new place is still on and Jane's still nagging to patch up."

I chose my words carefully so as not to hurt her, "You seem to be lonely."

Michele replied, "You are right, I am! You know, generally, I put up a façade, but I think I don't need to, here. It feels good to have one place at least where I can shed tears and 'be myself' without fabricating emotions."

We explored more on her feeling of loneliness, and how this break-up was different from the earlier ones.

Michele continued, "Well, all this while I broke up due to communication problems or lack of understanding; and most of the time, the men broke up with me, not the other way round. I was always left with no choice but to accept it, because it was decided by the other person. With Jane, however, I broke up, which is so unlike me. I feel guilty for behaving this way, but what she did is beyond repair. Interestingly, in my earlier relationships I was never as happy and committed as I was with Jane."

"It's hard to lose relationships which add meaning to our lives. Jane was sort of your strength, no wonder it hit you so hard. I feel sorry that you have to go through this," I said empathetically.

Michele remarked that she had gone through worse situations at home. I was quiet, waiting for her to continue further.

She hesitantly started, "I always felt helpless and lonely during my childhood but was lured by other pleasant thoughts and life changed as I grew older. Simmons truly changed my life. I became optimistic and somewhat daring as well. It's funny that I wasn't so disturbed, as I'm now, when I first started getting attracted to women. Now I feel sad though because it seems I'm quite unlucky as none of my relationships last long."

I clarified that breaking up with partners had nothing to do with self-worth, especially when Jane was at fault in this case.

Michele remained neutral and added, "Perhaps she wasn't happy with me and therefore became interested in Dory."

"What makes you think you were not good enough for her, or that her infidelity is because you lack something?"

"I don't know," she continued, "Negativity surrounds me whenever things go wrong. Maybe you are right, the problem lies with her, but how do I stop blaming myself? It's terrible!"

As I was thinking about her childhood, Michele interrupted, "Maybe you are right. I do tend to hold myself responsible for all the negatives that happen to me. It been this way ever since…I don't remember how long, my childhood probably!"

I asked if she wanted to share that part of her childhood.

"Full of nasty memories!" Michele exclaimed, "My earliest memories of childhood are all about fights; my parents fought almost every night which made our relationships quite dysfunctional. Most nights instead of lullabies, music and affection, I heard accusations, bickering and incessant quarrels. Often Mom would throw crockery on the kitchen floor, the sound grated on my ears. I would clutch Emily's arms and shut my eyes tightly."

"How old were you?," I asked.

"Oh well! It was all through my junior and high school."

On an optimistic note, I urged her to explore memories that were not as bitter, to which she commented, "Even if I had good days, I don't remember them much. In my efforts to maintain a balance between my parents, the negatives were so prevalent that they overshadowed all the positive points. Initially, I had to cope with my parents and their ongoing favouritism towards Emily, and then in school I had to be 'like others' so as to be included in the group."

I interupted, "Like whom?"

"I mean…. like the other girls, hiding all my attraction towards girls", Michele continued, "Life has been full of pretences for me."

I questioned further, "What'll happen if you let go off all your pretences and be yourself, the true Michele, inside and out?"

She looked at me and shook her head strongly, "No! I feel

vulnerable to do so. Everyone would know I am a lesbian and make fun of me, even my parents wouldn't support me."

Silence filled the room for a while after this statement.

"Well, Emily is the only one in whom I can confide," she attempted to explain, "We share the strongest of relationships that sisters can have. Though younger than I, she takes care of me more than Mom. Her affection overshadows Mom's indifferent behaviour when I visit home. She is the only meaningful relationship I have."

I interrupted, "Michele, you touched upon a lot of sensitive issues today, hope it won't manifest in any sort of depression or anxiety."

She laughed wryly. "Not yet, maybe when I grow old. You seem quite concerned, hope it's all genuine."

I immediately asked, "What made you think I might be faking?"

She instantly felt embarrassed, "I certainly didn't mean it that way. I think I have difficulty in accepting care and affection; there's always a fear of being betrayed."

"It's natural to feel depressed, especially since you have been hurt repeatedly under different circumstances, but there's no harm in being optimistic in life. Also, optimism should be intrinsic to your thoughts; though I'm glad you could express your thoughts here without filtering them."

Michele patiently listened and ended, "Optimism scares me, because whenever I feel so, I am betrayed. Moreover, the possibilities of heartbreak are less if I'm already thinking pessimistically. You know, it's like I have nothing to fear because there is nothing to lose!"

I was a bit awed by her explanation and thought no one ever

viewed pessimism so optimistically!! "You mean optimistic approach to life is risky?"

"Certainly, that's the way I feel! I know it's not a very healthy state of mind but it helps me to cope with the downside of my life."

She was in a vulnerable state of mind so I lightly mentioned, "Well! We could work on options to gear you up towards an optimistic attitude. The fact that you realize this is not a healthy way of thinking is the first step towards positive thinking."

Shortly after we finished our session, I fetched myself a glass of water and leant back in my chair with my eyes shut as her words rewound in my mind. My process of learning to detach myself from my clients' concerns and issues was not complete: the close connection that I felt tired me out mentally. I understood Michele's pain but could not imagine how it was to grow up within a discordant family.

I verbally ran over my thoughts about Michele's and was glad she felt comfortable to "be herself" within the counselling room. Her gestures and remarks made it clear that she was venting a lot of her bitter feelings and frustrations. She was sweating throughout, in spite of the moderate airconditioning, as she recounted her childhood. Sadly enough, she could not recall even one pleasant memory and insisted being comfortable with the negative thoughts. During childhood all through her growing years, she was subjected to constant parental fights and sibling comparison, because of which it seems she might be feeling incompetent and deem herself accountable for anything wrong that happens. If I wondered about her growing years contributing to such self-blame and low self-worth. Michele could accept her sexual identity, but it would require many more sessions before that.

I left the centre for the train-stop. The huddles of students, commuters, nagging children, pretty ladies and a lot more interesting people made the place colourful. I boarded the train but could not get a seat. As the train picked up speed, I gazed at the mid-sections of the pine trees which were visible through the square glass windows. They appeared spectacular, standing tall in rows and swaying sideways to the humming breeze. The sun had hidden behind the clouds and it was getting duller by the minute. When I got off the train, the sky was amber-orange with swathes of grey cutting through the endless limits. I thought if I were to sketch my mind, it would have probably looked the same, shades of grey of my thoughts running in different directions, interspersed with orange sparks of hope and optimism.

****

Later that night, I sat down to conceptualize Michele's life as much as I had known thus far. I knew Michele to be a survivor of childhood vulnerabilities, of betrayal and derogation, a victim of self-blame and guilt. Yet, I knew another side of Michele, a girl who was open to experimentation in life, striving for her independence and freedom. Michele was also a sincere client, a loving sister and a compliant daughter.

She had broken down because of her recent break-up, which sapped her mental strength and eroded her support system drastically; it brought back unpleasant memories of her childhood as well. Jane had sustained Michele through some of her confusions about herself with which she had been struggling previously. However, now that support was lost. I aspired to bring out the true person lurking inside her. I wanted to assist Michele to assert her own self, to listen to her heart, to live without fear or being dependent on someone.

****

It was late when I finished writing. It was dark outside and nothing was distinguishable from the window in front of my desk, except my own reflection on the glass pane. The hovering black clouds made the night seem darker than usual or perhaps I felt so after writing about Michele's dark experiences. My eyes felt heavy as I hit the sack, and I instantly fell asleep, travelling to dreamland within no time.

****

Memories—A Mixed Bag

Some things, as our memories, remain unmoved forever.
Joy, pain, fear and sorrow, our everlasting audience,
continually witnesses them

The following week, I spoke to Dr Sparks about all my clients, especially Amy whose binge eating sporadically escalated. She thought the same as I, that to comprehend her present, I had to delve into her childhood experiences. Dr Sparks also pointed on the importance of unconditional acceptance and empathy, especially during the times that Amy felt rejected.

The following day it was raining heavily before Michele's time slot, I was unsure if she would make it to the centre. The light drizzle had increased in intensity into almost a storm and the pitter-patter of the rain drops against the window pane became louder. The sky was partially visible from where I sat, and looked duller and darker than the usual August afternoons. I decided to wait for another couple of minutes for her and then start for home, before the bad weather got worse.

22 August, 2003

Session: 7

It was only our seventh session and my acquaintance with Michele attained new heights. She walked in five minutes late. I noticed her attire, which was unlike what she usually wore; she was partially drenched. She was fond of ethnic-style skirts and dresses with dangling earrings and slightly bold eye make-up; this time, it was denim jeans with a long-sleeved black shirt, and no jewellery or make-up, as if in mourning. Was it another form of self-punishment? I wondered.

I did not comment, lest it should make her feel conscious. Instead, I waited for her to say something to start the conversation. Michele greeted me–her voice sounded hoarse; I wondered if she had a cold or had been crying. Michele looked straight into my eyes, as if yearning to disclose something but could not. To put her at ease, I reminded her to speak her heart without being conscious.

Michele spoke after a little while, "I don't remember exactly where to start. It is hard switching back and forth everyday to the memories of the past."

I agreed but there was not much that I could offer without exploring her past; therefore I clarified, "The most difficult part in therapy is revisiting unfinished issues, traumatic incidents or childhood unpleasantness. I don't intend to force you with any topic; we could talk about something else today, if that suits you better."

By now she seemed a bit settled and replied, "Thanks for understanding! Actually I submitted a semester paper today, which had kept me awake last night. Feeling a bit drowsy! Besides, there has been stuff going on which I want to share with you."

I eagerly nodded indicating to her to continue.

"Finally this weekend," Michele began, "I am going to move out at last. I don't know how it'll be. I've never lived all by myself, but I think it's better than being with someone you can't stand."

"You may find it exciting to exercise your own choices. Where are you exactly moving to?"

'"This place is close to Simmons across the Fenway Park Street, also convenient from the train-stop and the Shaw's Grocery."

I was happy for her. "I guess you're all set to explore your new life then," I remarked.

"Right now I am simply glad to stick to my words or Jane would have thought I was pretending to leave. I even paid a month's rent in advance, just in case the landlord changed his mind. I am hoping it'll be for good and allow me time to introspect."

I added, "Since you mentioned about introspection, that might ensure some clarity of thoughts. Physical independence in turn would enable your mental independence, free from the constraints of conforming to others; a time to know yourself better as to who truly Michele is. At some point of time, we all need this space to liberate ourselves and to explore our desires, fears, innermost strengths and so forth."

Michele responded, attending to my suggestions, "Talking to you undeniably clarifies my thoughts and fortifies me with optimism."

"Thanks indeed! I am glad it's helpful."

Michele spoke some more about her new accommodation before we switched gears to discuss her family's reaction to this change.

"As expected, they are not accepting it as a positive thing.

Mom feels this would ruin my career as I would indulge in 'wrong' relationships and waste time and eventually mess up academically. She is not aware of my experience with Jane. It's weird, because she doesn't realize that I can party living with roommates also!"

I commented, "So how are you thinking of handling it?"

There was indifference in her voice as she spoke, "We are not on talking terms. I called her last night to let her know about my plans and the new address; but she hung up on me and my Dad never bothered either."

"It must be hurting that your Dad doesn't care?"

Michele laughed self-deprecatingly and said, "I'll be surprised if he knew my course and college's name properly!! It's been this way ever since my childhood. I've got accustomed to it by now. Mom fought with him often because of his negligence towards us, his home and family. She even spied on Dad through her friends, to know if he was seeing someone. Fortunately, it never yielded positive results."

"It seems your parents were quite engrossed in resolving their own differences. It must have been hard, at times, feeling neglected."

She remained silent for a while and then spoke, "What choice did I have? Emily was too young to understand all this stuff, Dad never had time and Mom was mad at me for almost everything. I did get attention, but it was negative."

Description of Michele's family was typically dysfunctional, showing lack of communication where parents curbed the growth of their children; and constant bickering further deteriorated the situation. Exploring some more I inquired, "Did you make conscious efforts to please them, to be in their good books?"

"Yes, it is true that I've always tried, though I never succeeded to get their love and affection. If they know my sexual orientation, I will never get their love or approval ever in life. You know, sometimes I feel cursed, as to why it happened to me, why am I not like Emily or my other friends; why was I born to such parents?"

We were in the middle of an emotional moment. I imagined myself in her place and felt her misery. "Why do you think your lesbian identity will worsen the relationship?"

"I know it will! Homosexuality is unacceptable in my family. Mom once commented that if same-sex marriages aren't banned, our society will be in shambles. Besides, she openly loathed my lesbian friends in school whom she knew. A gay couple had moved in our complex and my Mom got angry at the landlord for letting out accommodation to them. I mean, she's quite irrational when it comes to equality and open-mindedness."

"It seems you are preparing yourself to face the worst," I contemplated, "Time is the best healer; it manages things which we can't settle ourselves. Your mother might require more time to accept the truth. Start talking to her so that at least you are in touch." She stared at me blankly as if I spoke a different language, "You are mentioning a dream! I wish my Mom was ready to talk; but her mood swings mostly rule our conversation. Maybe, a visit in the near future would help, since she can't avoid me at home. However, I'm not considering all this now; no added stress from Mom is needed. I already have enough to handle."

"I'm hoping it will be soon!" Then, hesitantly Michele excused herself, "Is it okay if I leave a bit early today? There are a few books I have to return to the library." I willingly affirmed her departure, "I'll see you next week; all the best for your new place."

Michele walked out and Rene entered with a new case history for me. I kept the new case aside while I finished Michele's process notes. Her vulnerability had become evident, especially when she stated her mother's attitude towards homosexuality. Michele's thoughts, words, and expressions pervaded the room as I wrote.

Process notes: 7

Michele is somewhat anxious about this decision but expects that it will provide her the freedom she has always longed for. I contemplated on her mother's perspective and thought maybe she had a valid point; but given the strained relationship Michele shared with her mother I reassured that it was normal to feel stressed until she was able to reconcile her mind. She is quite convinced that her family, especially her mother, will never approve of her lesbian identity, as it would derogate their social status. Though she is not considering disclosing this issue to her parents now, it seems to haunt her mind repeatedly.

****

By the time I walked out of the centre, it was almost deserted and had started getting dark outside. The train was not so crowded and I managed to get a seat; while I did so, two adorable little girls caught my attention. They were probably between the age of four to six, and were giggling and playing with their hair and comparing their arms and fidgeting with their fancy little bags. One of them was White, while the other had dark skin. Their mother, seated next to them, was White. I assumed their father was probably African-American. The girls were busy in their own unaffected play-world.

I speculated how it would be when the two grow up, especially for the dark-skinned girl. Soon they skipped down from the train, clutching their mother's fingers. I did not know them nor would I ever see them again. However, I can still recall their faces and think about the little dark-skinned girl.

In my opinion, skin tone had nothing to do with romantic attraction as such. Nonetheless some men still prefer their better half to be fair skinned, especially in India. I often found it hilarious while flipping through the matrimonial columns in the newspaper, where consistently all the eligible brides were described as fair and good looking. I wondered if lesbian woman also felt similarly.

****

In our following session, Michele was 20 minutes early for our eighth session. I found her pacing in the reception on the way to my office. I requested Rene to ask her to wait until her usual time slot, because there was some urgent work which I had to finish before the session.

29 August, 2003

Session: 8

Michele immediately started about her new place as soon as she entered the room. "I really like it! The apartment is less spacious compared to the previous one, but for a single person, it's perfect. I've been spending my days and nights quiet peacefully without my interferences. Last weekend I even invited some friends over for supper; it was good fun and I am also able to concentrate better on my studies." While speaking suddenly her voice became softer and trailed off. She became silent in the middle of the session, her cheeks went red and tears rolled down. She was unable to speak.

"Michele, are you alright? What happened?"

"It's the same old problem! Mom has nothing better than to poke her nose in my life. On Wednesday I went out to dinner with Becky, one of my classmates. Unknowingly, I left my mobile at home. Mom called up several times that night, to check on me, and supposedly became worried. Later, when I spoke to her she was furious and accused me unnecessarily."

"She seems to overreact on trivial matters," I concurred.

Michele nodded and kept weeping, "Exactly! Once Dad was about to leave home because of her nagging and accusations. After a furious fight over some seemingly unimportant matter, Dad warned her not to irritate him, but she kept on going. He lost his temper and threw a ceramic vase placed at the corner table at the wall and declared he had tolerated enough. I think my prayers were heard that day and he decided to stay back. I still shiver when I recall that evening."

As much as I tried, I could not imagine myself in such situation because I was not brought up in such an environment. Michele proclaimed facing worst experiences than this. "Many nights, I remember, Dad never returned home, probably slept with other women. It wasn't that Mom was ignorant of his acts, but she continued to put up with him, knowing all his shortcomings. She would sulk all day and all night until we became the target of her anger, mostly me. As I grew older, I understood more of their slanging matches. My hunch about my Dad's extramartial affairs clearly became evident later."

She sobbed incessantly recalling those days. Then she tried to control herself and continued, "I couldn't comprehend why Mom never left Dad when she had all the reasons. She often attended phone calls from unknown women for my Dad while he was away. Those nights she hardly ate or slept. She would throw things around in a fit of extreme anger and cry uncontrollably in her room and then magically, when Dad returned home in the morning, as if nothing happened. Her resentment was manifest only before us, her daughters. I knew she loathed my Dad but never showed it; maybe she feared that he would abandon her and she couldn't have raised us without Dad's financial support. She was probably in a fix! Sometimes I blame myself. Why was I even born? Had I not been there, maybe she could have managed the expenses of one child, Emily, and left Dad, living her life independently. Guilt haunts me often…."

I was silent.

"You've handled pretty rough experiences at a very tender age. I'm sorry to hear about your parents' relationship and the way it affected you. But there is no reason to blame yourself. Did you ever try to commit any self-destructive behaviour?"

"No never. But I do blame myself often because I think he only reason Mom stuck with Dad was because of us I wonder if she ever secretly wished me dead or something, maybe my presence was unwanted, which is why she found fault in everything I did…till date. It may be my assumption, but Mom's indifference towards me makes it believable."

"Lack of communication may have led to such feelings," I said.

It seemed she was not convinced about lack of communication but she did not contradict me either. "Also, when I was about 12 or 13, Mom began restricting our food choices. All her life she's been quite figure-conscious. She went to such extremes that she never allowed us even a piece of cake or chocolate. She reasoned it would be embarrassing to have plump daughters."

"Was your Mom ever plump?"

"Yes she was, but she reduced tremendously and is still in shape," Michele responded. "She had a horror of being overweight and did not want us to be obese. It was not just a restriction on junk food but all food. She would limit the quantity and, of course, let us have only what she thought was appropriate. On some nights, for dinner she would give us only salad; my Dad, of course, never bothered about what we ate or rather, what we did not. He was only concerned with his meals. We used to creep down to the kitchen after she had gone to bed and forage for anything to eat. My Dad was fond of cookies, so despite Mom's protests, he used to keep a stash of them. Emily and I used to often steal cookies and eat in our room. It was not unusual to lie awake because of the growling in our stomachs. Mom caught us once while grabbing cookies. She punished us on that account and berated me for being greedy. She gave me nothing to eat and I remained hungry for nearly the whole of the next morning. She relented only when Dad protested."

"That's terrible!" I exclaimed. Generally I never reacted this way, expressing my own feelings or taking a client's side; but her experiences made it hard to remain neutral.

Michele had been speaking in a monotone, as if any expression would overwhelm her. Pausing briefly she continued, "Somehow Mom never got infuriated much with Emily, maybe because of her age. I always had to bear the brunt of her rage, being the older one."

"Even now, although both of us are away from home, Mom cares more for Emily. This is nothing new. But revisiting my childhood is painful. I think the fact that Emily and I are so close disturbs Mom."

Michele was deeply disturbed recounting her childhood as she thought aloud, "Honestly, I've seen her at her worst during my childhood. Maybe, that's the reason I fear history being repeated again if I disclose my secret to Mom."

I sensed her mounting anxiousness and advised her not to panic. "Take things one at a time, as it comes. Be easy on yourself."

Michele agreed, "I know I tend to get very anxious and tense–I try not to, but can't help it! It is not easy to remain calm when things go wrong. I can't ignore the fact that Mom is not talking to me; but I can't change the situation either."

"I can understand it's hard to remain calm, especially, when you have such unresolved differences. How about contacting your Mom through emails? Do you think that'll work? I don't intend to take sides; but maybe she's concerned about your safety as you are living alone. Her anger might be a form of expressing her concern."

She clarified her reactions to the various situations in a rational manner despite the emotional turbulence that had been evoked. Since we were already nearing the end of our session, there was no point in introducing fresh aspects at this juncture.

At the end of the session I inquired, "How was your experience of sharing such disturbing accounts, memories of which were buried deep?" "It wasn't easy; I almost felt it was a replay of my childhood. Actually, it's more of an internal suffocation which I feel."

I sat alone, thinking, for long after she had left. I could not imagine how it was to be raised in an environment such as she had described. There was nothing in common between us; but still, I felt close to her pain and apprehensions.

Some days my clients made my heart sink; this was one of those days. I contemplated to myself; tears are often the most meaningful medium of expression. They can convey more than words, and sometimes, one could construe a whole new world from them. Though this was not the first time that Michele had shed tears, but the intensity of her sorrow filled the room. Clearly, Michele's present instability in relationships was somewhat a pronounced influence of her childhood insecurities. I felt a lump in my throat; her sufferings made me tearful. The time we sat in silence as the session wound down was unlike the silence we shared in the beginning sessions.

The room, which was my office, had witnessed heart-wrenching sorrows and experiences; never-before mentioned truths, confessions and desires of people who were unknown till they sat in the chair opposite me. It was also a silent witness to the evolution of an apprehensive novice counsellor on the threshold of her career.

****

Good Thoughts Chase Away Bad Times

Life is slipping by every minute,
rejuvenate it with nothing but optimism

I had been out since morning on Sunday. After finishing my overtime hours at Starbucks, I headed straight to the library. By the time I returned home, it was late evening. The 100-year-old house, then my temporary abode, stood sturdy against the windy evening. I unlocked the main entrance door and found Patty's blue-eyed cat, Rasky, who greeted me with his lazy "meows". There was a wicker chair in the porch, in which he used to curl up and snooze through the day. Patty must have put him inside as the evening was windy. I was alone that evening with Rasky for company. The family occasionally went out for late-night movies on weekends. Shelby often accompanied them. Patty had offered me to come along as well but due to my timings I couldn't make it.

The rugs placed on the wooden floors in the living room looked dull from the imprint of countless footprints. I switched on the lights that Patty was so fond of, while Rasky followed me soundlessly. He bounded ahead of me when I turned towards the kitchen, mewing in anticipation. He reminded me of the fat men of ancient times, who did nothing but sit on silken cushions and eat all day long.

I opened the fridge, which was filled with the mixed aromas of Italian, Chinese and Indian food. The top shelf generally contained organic 1 per cent milk and soyamilk, juices and Hershey's chocolate syrup. Salads always found its place in a bowl or two. Vegetables, which mostly I bought, comprised cherry tomatoes, mushrooms, green beans and lettuce, were on the lowest shelf. Patty and her daughters, as well as Shelby, mostly lived on frozen and canned foods, and occasional home-cooked meals.

My dinner was simple and I ate it while surfing the television channels. There was nothing interesting to watch. Moreover, I was too exhausted to sit through the programmes. I seconded the entrance lock and went upstairs to my room. Rasky did not follow me. He used to sometimes sleep outside my room by the door. But one night I tripped over him in the dark on my way to the bathroom and nearly squashed him. After that, he kept to the ground floor at night.

****

I snuggled in my bed, which was then the most luxurious moment of the day! This was the time when I thought randomly of various things, made tentative plans.

I thought how it would be returning to India. My friends from India often called through the internet and we chatted for hours.

That truly felt good, as if I was connected back to old world of happenings.

My thoughts returned back to Boston and it was my clients who enticed me the most. I thought about the trust my clients had reposed in me, to become a part of their world, of "knowing", would not have been possible in India. I thought of many things besides my clients. Simmons had given me the opportunity to interact with people whom I considered far different from what I was familiar to me. I was learning to retain myself "in the moment" with clients without losing my own views. Counselling–as I began evolving–essentially presented to me a world that intrigued and engrossed me completely. I drifted off to sleep thinking of these things.

While writing Michele's process notes, I realised that she had become one of my favourite clients, not only because of her punctuality or her cordial behaviour, but simply because we connected well. Nothing, as a counsellor, was more rewarding for me than to gain the confidence and trust of my clients. My empathy towards her had been augmented, maybe because of the conviction in our bonding.

5 September, 2003

Session: 9

By the ninth session I knew Michele would be able to withstand difference of opinion or minor confrontations in sessions if required.

She wore a black halter-neck top with blue denims, her hair was loose which cascaded over her shoulders, while the antique earrings completed the look perfectly. Her face was glowing and she had her usual smile, which had vanished over the past few weeks. I assumed things were proceeding well.

"Hi there, I'm actually doing pretty well this week; and like always, have loads to fill you up on."

I exclaimed, "That's right, you sound cheerful!"

Michele excitedly followed, "Well, I think I am! I have recently met someone. We are just good friends as of now, her name's Rachael. I wouldn't say I'm in love, but I enjoy her company. She is a sophomore in the English department."

"It seems you feel secure when you are with someone."

"True! It's really easy when I hear you speak my mind," she added. "I've noticed since past few weeks, especially after sharing my childhood experiences, that I feel quite comfortable sharing anything and everything during sessions. It's like now I've let myself free and there's nothing to be ashamed of or to hide."

I appreciated her thoughts. "I think it's extremely commendable that you are able to open up and discuss all ups and downs without any inhibitions. There isn't any reason to belittle yourself just because your Mom or some other person rejects you! Live for the present; no one is gifted with a perfect life. It depends on what we do to make it perfect." Michele mumbled hesitantly, "Even when I try to be happy, my past troubles haunt me. I often compromise on my own pleasures in the process of pleasing others."

"Do you feel valued only through positive feedback from others?" I questioned.

"Perhaps maybe," she continued, "A note of appreciation always makes my day."

"That's true for all of us, but does your happiness depend on that solely?"

I explored more, "How would you define happiness in your life?"

There was a brief silence. "Well, I am not sure if I can answer that precisely. Happiness to me is enjoying life in a way that everyone loves me. Sometimes, just being myself also feels good, like the way I am here." She laughed softly and continued, "Optimism and support from others always scores high in my list of happiness."

I interjected, "And that adds to a feeling of completeness."

"Sort of," she replied, raising her eyebrows.

"In the last couple of minutes, everything you said had to do with pleasing others or regarding their perception towards you. However, I missed hearing about what brings happiness to Michele irrespective of others' viewpoints."

Michele stared at me blankly

"I may have evoked too many disturbing thoughts; is it hard to accept all this in one go?"

"No-not at all! I was quiet because your question shook me; no one has asked me this before."

"Then you must have lots to reflect on," I began. "Actually self-reflection and introspection is required at every stage of life. It makes one decide one's own choices and take responsibility for one's own actions."

"I am trying to reflect; but truly the happiest thing for me would be if Mom praises me someday. It'll be truly meaningful, but I can't see it happening in near future. Instead it's getting worse by the week."

Instead of reassuring her with platitudes, I guided her thoughts productively, "Make efforts towards evolving concrete strategies on enhancing communication skills with your Mom. You might have to make efforts to take the initial step, but eventually they might bring in some positive results."

Michele abruptly changed track and she exclaimed, "I am thinking of another thing that fills me with happiness, it's dancing!" Her face brightened instantly. "I loved it as a child and still do. I remember dancing to the latest tracks in front of the mirror while growing up but Mom considered it as indecent. I was often lectured on manners and proper behaviour subsequent to my dancing."

I ventured deeper, "Did you ever feel like revolting when your mother accused you?"

"Yes I did!" she remarked embarrassingly. "I regret not being bold enough to stand up for myself and do what made me joyous; I gave up dancing completely, hoping that some day she would appreciate my obedience and let me dance."

"And you are still waiting...?," I let my voice trail away.

Michele quietly nodded. Gazing through the window she resumed, "Sometimes I feel tired of pleasing others. It hampers my own individuality, but I don't know how to break through. Maybe it's too late now, because now if I attend to my own decisions, others might find me rude or arrogant. You see, everyone's so accustomed to my compliance."

I smiled, "Tricky, is it? Do you realize how habits almost become our second identity?"

"That's right, never thought about it though!" she said surprised at this insight.

"However, nothing is impossible, it may take time but it's never too late to assert your individuality. Besides, the 'others' that you are concerned about will get accustomed to the 'new' you. Who are these 'others' and why must you fear their opinion?"

"Well, it's easier said than done, I think," she said hesitantly.

"Certainly, I don't intend to sound like a teacher, instructing you good and bad rather it's just an option, if you wish to change yourself, never be afraid to embark on it." I added, "Once you start respecting yourself, your needs, likes and dislikes, you will be more in control of your life as well. Seemingly small changes often go a long way in fortifying life with optimism."

At last, she asked thoughtfully, "Like I love to dance, so should I join classes now, as no one ever encouraged me to do so earlier? Is that asserting my wishes?"

I appreciated her promptness. "Sure, it sounds like a great idea. Any form of art relaxes the mind and you might make new friends and expand your circle beyond Simmons."

This time the session ended on an optimistic note and was more constructively than the previous ones. It marked yet another turning point in the counselling process.

****

I started for home. The wind outside had no intentions of settling, while I crossed the twisting and turning pathways towards the main road. Everything seemed so vibrant and bright; truly, autumn was the most colourful of all seasons. Soon the colours, along with all the leaves, would wither away leaving behind a monochrome of the winter ahead. Walking past the Simmons dormitory, which was partially visible from the main road, I thought about my clients and their lives residing there. Once I even caught glimpse of Michele and Jane holding hands in a convenient store. Likely she hadn't noticed me and knowing she would be embarrassed I preferred not to greet her either. Then I was also new to the concept of lesbian love and found it somewhat uncomfortable to accept. With time, however, I began to realize that it was only a matter of personal liking, no big deal!

There were instances when I came across my clients in the store or at the train-station; the dilemma whether to smile or not always puzzled me. Some never bothered to recognize me in front of their partners or whoever accompanied them, while others would smile weakly. I respected both options fairly well as it was entirely their choice to deal with such situations. Had I been in their shoes, I might have reacted in a similar fashion as well. While travelling back I thought indepth about my clients, their extended families as I knew them and so forth.

When I got back home, I quickly slipped into a soothing shower and my warm corduroy pyjamas smelled so fresh and fragrant after washing it in the aromatic detergent.

I pushed aside the thoughts of pending work as I settled down to read, reading fiction in the safety of home away from the inclement weather outside felt cozy. However, after I began, I found it hard to concentrate after two or three pages. My mind kept racing back to the session with Michele. Today, there was chirpiness in her voice which boded well. Our session had marked a new beginning within our counsellor-client relationship. Owing to her comfort level, for the first time, I confronted Michele about her idea of happiness in terms of how she perceived it.

Michele recognizes that her own thoughts, wishes and desires are seldom regarded as a possibility and thus are neglected. In my opinion, she desired attention more because she was deprived of it from an early age. I had noted that even the most negligible amount of admiration or approval would make Michele's face glow. Her sense of achievement was dependent on the way others perceived her, to which she attributed her self-esteem and individuality, such dependency had possibilities of hampering her individuality.

****

The mornings had become chillier than before with the advent of September. The true colours of autumn were evident in the maple and mulberry trees never fail to charm the first-time visitors, and I was no exception. The shades of the leaves were very different and seemed magical. The riot of colours was something I had not seen before. Delhi has its share of colours too, the brilliant yellow of the amaltas competing with the early summer sun, the purple jacaranda, the pink of the kachnar and the fluffy white of the silk cotton during the short spring and the plethora of hues of the flowers in winter. But compared to this, what I had seen before seemed staid. Who knew autumn could be so enticing? It seemed as if nature had adorned herself with red, orange, yellow and amber-coloured jewels like the queens of yore. The ground too echoed some of the colour in the leaves which were blown off the branches by the wind and crunched underfoot as one walked.

In spite of being single I found myself feeling romantic witnessing the boundless beauty of the nature.

Although I used to have a hectic schedule all week, Fridays always seemed longer, strenuous and too loaded. I could hardly steal some time for myself. I was beginning to understand clients more profoundly beyond the literal meaning of what they shared with me. It fetched me a lot of knowledge in counselling through opportunities to experience vicariously through various clients' lives.

12 September, 2003

Session: 10

On this day, Michele started right away as if she had been waiting for this moment to blurt out her feelings. "I've been thinking a lot about our previous session all this week. You know it's amazing, the more I thought, the deeper it drew me within."

"Could you elaborate a bit on that?"

Michele continued, 'It's all interrelated I presume! I'm talking about becoming more assertive, like you had mentioned in the previous session, to boost my self-esteem and confidence. Ever since I became aware of how I always was seeking approval, I feel like a loser. Honestly, I don't want to feel this way any longer. It started with conforming to Mom's wishes to keep her happy, and then the pattern continued with friends and in now relationships as well. It is draining."

I asked, "Now when you view your past behavioural patterns do you really feel like a loser?"

Michele affirmed my words, "I do, but now I am going to give value to my own wishes and desires, which I couldn't, for instance, dancing. At least I'll try to join because no one encouraged me to do so, even Jane thwarted me. You are the first person to mention this and bring forth this thought last week. In spite of being reasonably good at it, I never gave a second thought about pursuing dancing as it was not appreciated by those who mattered to me."

She paused and continued, "How to actually go about altering my habit of pleasing others? Those who know me well have seldom known the other side of me. Wouldn't it be odd to voice my opinions suddenly, how will they react to it?"

"Who are the 'they' that you are concerned about?," I queried.

Michele remained silent. Perhaps she did not know herself who the "they" were.

However, I reaffirmed her doubts, "I know it sounds audacious but that's what you need to do. Initially this transition might seem difficult but it'll enhance your confidence in the long run."

She asked doubtfully, "Don't you think such behaviour can make me unpopular and lose friendships?"

"Yes it might, to start with, do you think that's reason enough to let go of your own wishes and conform to others?"

Michele was confused momentarily, "I …I don't know, but yes I am definitely apprehensive about asserting my feelings, thoughts, and likewise. Although I know this would allow me to exercise my choices freely, the fear of rejection by others is a constant."

"I feel the more we explore, you'll find it easier to accept yourself within this new framework."

"Yes, that's something I really need to work on because most of my thoughts are governed by others. Being a follower is easier! Now, with a new beginning though I am looking forward to reinvent myself."

Michele countered immediately, "My dating relationships are hidden and no one would know even if things went wrong, not even my Mom, but altering my habits or behaviour is way more challenging."

Our conversation now took a significant turn then. I was excited that Michele questioned and responded assertively when I probed. I finally shared my insight with her. "It seems you fear taking responsibilities on an explicit level, but feel at ease if it's private, like your relationships or like our counselling sessions."

Her eyes glistened as she looked at me with surprise, "Did I ever exercise my choices in here?"

I will never forget the expression on Michele's face that moment. It was as if a million stars had kissed her skin.

"Yes indeed you did just now by contradicting my opinions. So, I want you to consider that if you can do it in private situations, then why fear experimenting a bit openly? Also you have to 'come out' to your family and friends at some point of time. Would you deny your desires and your partner then, for the sake of others?," I asked pointedly.

"I never thought about it. My reaction was rather a spontaneous reaction to your suggestion. Nevertheless, I'm glad it happened and probably at the safest place possible," she replied, still recovering from the insightful thought.

All of a sudden, Michele's voice again began to tremble and

sounded hoarse as she explained, "I was never popular in school, enjoying a gang of friends or something, till today my groups of friends are quite numbered. Among many other factors one of the prominent reasons for this is because I'm a lesbian. Now, if I start responding the way you suggested, I might just repel even my limited group of friends. I fear being lonely again; it reminds me of my miserable childhood." The silence lingered longer than expected. I was assimilating the course of the session. Her slightly uncompromising tone informed me that she was confronting my thoughts for the second time. This time she was firmer than before.

Once more like before, I summed up the session as it ended that day, "It seems you have pushed yourself to become more self-assertive. I'll be glad to see you respond this way more often. Also, don't let go all your support at once, referring back to your concern. Be assertive about some of the choices, if not all to begin with. Be optimistic, that'll change your outlook and handle some of your fear as well."

Her eyes showed that she felt good as she walked away. I felt contented; my efforts had begun to yield fruit. I could not wait to jot down the proceedings of the session in my office itself.

Process notes: 10

I feel therapy is showing beneficial results, especially since the last two sessions. I am witnessing subtle changes within Michele from her first session with me to this session. Her new-found vision added to Michele's awareness. I knew she felt scared to own responsibilities, but had begun to take fairly significant decision independently as well. Also, I noticed that Michele tried to settle matters by the end of each session. It could have been her way of gaining control over her life.

After each process note that I wrote, I felt a surge of strength within me. There was so much to learn and reflect on, on the basis of my clients' lives, it continually intrigued me. Given our discrepant backgrounds and childhood experiences, Michele entirely transformed my approach and attitude towards homosexuality and rendered me more liberal. At some level, I envied her strength to withstand all odds alone, and it certainly demanded respect.

Academics bore the brunt of this struggle as I started devoting more time to my clientele and internship. However, I was not the only one in that situation; several of my classmates were placed similarly. Not only did I counsel them but also learnt aspects about my own stereotypical perceptions. I wondered if other amateur counsellors also felt the same with some of their clients.

As the months progressed, it became imperative that I manage my schedule efficiently. No doubt that it was stressful, but was pretty satisfying at the same time. It was beginning to get challenging to strike a balance between personal and professional life.

Well personal life became so limited that they remained mostly in thoughts. We were a group of three–me, Amanda and Teri. It was always fun hanging out with my girlfriends, though time was a real constraint. Teri was completing her internship at a children's hospital due to which her timings did not quite match ours. Amanda was placed at another college counselling setting, similar to mine, which made it convenient for us to plan outings. Amanda's boyfriend was French who was pretty demanding, most of the evenings she would spend with him as much time as she could.

Weekends were always a real treat. I usually started my day at the crack of dawn, heading out for a stroll near the riverside, roughly about 10 minutes' walk from Patty's place. The fresh nippy air had traces of the September chill which was becoming more and more apparent. The quiet moments as I walked through the woods offered solitude which used to recharge me for the day ahead. Undoubtedly physically I always felt fresh but mentally I often missed the presence of someone special in my life. Especially when I saw couples sharing their good times together.

The weekend that followed was the beginning of the advent of fall colours. It was sunny, generously spreading its brightness, devoid of any wet spells. Neighbourhood parks served as the meeting point for all. Children indulged in their favourite sports while adults chose to dress skimpily, lie in the sun and tan themselves. It never failed to amuse me that I, who belonged to the race of the 'original' sun worshippers, would shudder at the prospect of exposing myself to the September chill in a similar fashion; and would scurry indoors when it was warmer. Young, muscular men wore branded shorts but were bare-chested, occupied a significant portion of the park and played basketball. A few loners enjoyed reading or sipped drinks and celebrated their weekend. The park was a joyous place which was on the way to the grocer. Occasionally, friends would accompany me for grocery shopping, but not on this weekend.

I walked past the Jewish synagogue on Beacon Street. People were gathered at the entrance, laughing and gossiping. Women accompanied by dapperly dressed men, couples holding hands, pretty little girls dressed in lace frocks and little boys in their smart outfits, lingered in front of it. Perhaps there was a wedding that morning. This was the second time I witnessed a wedding. A cluster of women indulged in some rituals and were singing softly, probably a Jewish wedding song. I felt happy for the soon-to-be-wed couple, though I caught only a glimpse of them. The bride looked gorgeous in her wedding attire. She seemed somewhat taller than the groom. I laughed to myself because Indian women mostly preferred their men to be taller than them. In the US, however, I had seen quite a few couples vice-versa, it wasn't a big issue. I loved noticing these little cultural deviations. It was a pleasant deviation from my usual routine as I headed further to the grocer's.

The stores in the US were truly a feast for the eyes and light on the pocket as well. The first time I visited one in Rochester, I was awed with the endless varieties and choices. Unlike India, here the food and other necessary items were at affordable prices for everyone; a plumber or car washer as well as a company executive. One could also indulge in moderate luxuries, once in a while. I wished fervently that someday India, too, would be able to provide the basic requirement to all its citizens.

There were elaborate selections of milk, from soyamilk to full cream, organic to lactose-free; an endless assortment of cookies; sugar-free, real or artificial fruit juices and jams. There was a wide selection of cheese; some new ones that I discovered were Blue Cheese and Gruyere Cheese. Fruits and vegetables in myriad colours were neatly stacked. It felt like a magic house where one was spoiled for choice. The list was endless and this was only a local grocer; imagine the country-wide chains!

I picked up some vegetables, fruits, a few "heat-n-eat" cans of kidney beans, black beans, chickpeas, a loaf of wholewheat cinnamon bread, which was a favourite of mine, a half-gallon carton of one per cent milk, a box of salted crackers, some tissues, a phone-card and two pencil batteries. By the time I stepped out of the store, it was windy and cloudy as the sun had disappeared behind them. Boston weather was more unpredictable than human nature!

****

A New Ray of Light

Live for today; let not fears of
the past haunt the present

The next session with Michele was quite interesting and entirely unexpected. That Friday is etched in my mind because of the tangential course on which the session proceeded.

19 September, 2003

Session: 11

It was cloudy and overcast; the client scheduled ahead of Michele had cancelled due to bad weather. I was not expecting Michele either, but she arrived, partly soaked in her denims and long-sleeved blue tee-shirt. Her blond hair looked like tangled wet golden threads. It had been raining cats and dogs for the last two days. The weekend was predicted to be damp and mildly chilly— it was definitely a time for family time together. I sorely missed mine on such days as it had been over six months since I had visited them.

Michele carried a brown paper bag containing a box of chocolates along with a small bouquet of carnations, which she placed beside her chair. A card slipped out of her bag which she handed over to me.

The card was embossed with pink roses, it read: "To Someone Special." I flipped it open and read, "Dear Michele," below it was a printed quotation on true friends. On the left side, Rachael had personalized it with her own handwriting.

"I have not known you since long but am glad that we met. This is the day we had first met, a month ago. Thank you for giving me so many beautiful reasons to smile and unforgettable moments. You hold a special place in my heart and always will. Though I've had many friendships before, there's a special bond I feel with you. No one has understood me the way you do. I am truly blessed to have you beside me to cry and laugh and to share the good and the not-so-good times.

Always with love, Rachael"

I appreciated Rachael's thoughts and handed the card back to Michele. Her eyes shone with contentment. She seemed happy unlike the past weeks. Michele urged me to comment about Rachael's card and her entire gesture of celebrating the anniversary of their month-old friendship. "It's wonderful that Rachael remembered and acknowledged the love she feels for you in such a special way. I am sure it means a lot to you. Did you reciprocate our feelings as well?," I asked. She smiled and then smiled some more. "Yeah, I feel like I am on cloud nine. I wished her but forgot to buy something special, maybe this evening we'll go out for a candle-light dinner. I know she'll love that!!"

"Sounds like a perfect plan! You both deserve to celebrate this moment," I added.

"As you know, all my previous relationships, neither sex ever gave me this feeling. This might sound bizarre, but I feel I'm in a trance; I fear waking up. Rachael has been the sweetest person I have known better than Jane. I hope it remains this way. Introspecting now, I feel maybe it was for the best that I broke up with Jane or else I wouldn't have met Rachael. It is true everything happens for a reason and in my case it's a very good reason." Her blue eyes, full of radiance and depth, made me to think that she was in love with Rachael.

"I'm sure she'll value your emotions and reciprocate similarly."

Michele agreed. "I hope so too, as a matter of fact," she lingered, "I'm waiting for Rachael to let me know if she has similar feelings as I do. On several occasions I hinted to her that I was interested in a serious relationship, but she was non-committal."

I probed further, "Is she aware of all your past relationships?"

"Yes, we confided in the other about our past. However, we soon became busy with each other and the past became secondary," Michele exclaimed elated.

"I wish I could share about Rachael with my family but I can't, except perhaps, with Emily, if at all. Coming out is like a nightmare."

"And you want to keep it closed forever?"

"Why is everything ruined just because I'm a lesbian?"

"It's ruined because you tend to judge all spheres of life, happiness and achievement in terms of this one factor. Unless you feel comfortable yourself, how will others accept you? They'll respect you only when you respect yourself."

She nodded. I was unsure whether she really understood or it was a mere acknowledgment of what I said.

"This time I won't repeat the same mistakes or let anyone walk over me like Jane. Emotional bonding is more important for me than getting physical." Michele dwelt on her last words for a couple of minutes and then softly murmured, "I can wait until Rachael is ready for it."

I noticed that this time she took the situation in her stride without rushing it, I tip-toed very lightly about how things were going with her Mom.

She instantly became pale, "I've been thinking of Mom lately. She always shatters my happy moments so I didn't talk to her. However, I spoke to Emily about Rachael and she seemed quite excited, like always."

"Emily's your one and only family support," I added.

"Absolutely," she agreed.

A strange but fairly significant incident happened following our conversation. Michele halted momentarily and commented, "There's one more person with whom I can be myself and that's you."

I was certainly not expecting this. I thanked her and affirmed warmly to her response. Michele's eyes were watery and I felt mine tearing up too. She wiped her tears with the pink tissues stacked inside the box. "I don't have a place to cry at home, but here I can be myself. It's cathartic. I'm able to vent out all my emotions and feelings without worrying about any consequences."

"Well, that's the beauty of counselling." I knew she needed a lot of unconditional support and acceptance.

"This is your space and I am here to listen to you. I appreciate your feedback."

Before leaving she commented, "It's weird that whenever I come for sessions I cry. Almost feels customary now! Can I ever leave this place without crying?" She laughed lightly; her eyes still watery and the kohl smudged around the corners.

"Michele!" I cried out, "Time will witness those moments too."

Unlike some of my other clients, Michele never dragged sessions unnecessarily. She inspired me as a counsellor by allowing counselling to unfold in innovative ways. I decided to transfer my thoughts on paper while travelling back to Boston College, lest I forget. I jotted the following:

Process notes: 11

Michele was extremely overjoyed, her eyes gleamed with optimism. There was nothing personal or professional about the situation, but I was more than pleased that she shared her good moments with me as well.

Michele urged me to endorse her friendship with Rachael. Being her counsellor, I presumed it added more validity to her thoughts somehow. She had the look of a little girl's anticipation, eager to hear her favourite story.

Despite her happiness, there was an undercurrent of insecurity and fear of losing Rachael. Counselling was the only space that allowed her to unfold her emotions and feelings without being conscious. I finished writing just in time before my stop arrived. It would be a week before I would see Michele; I looked forward to the session with eagerness.

****

The evening was dark and quiet as I headed towards Loveland Road. The sound of the chilly wind steadily rose above that of the swishing cars. I felt the tip of my nose and then my ears grow numb with cold. I pulled my hair over my ears, but it did not help. My fingers felt warm tucked inside the corduroy jacket. However, it was refreshing to be out in the fresh air after being in the central heating rooms all day long.

It was not very late when I reached home. Courtney was on the phone and Symphony was watching TV–this was something unusual because they were never at home. Perhaps Courtney had had a fight with her boyfriend, I thought.

After dinner, I wanted to watch a movie, but could not decide which one. Dropped that idea and called up a couple of friends in India and Houston. Gossiping was no less fun than a movie! My friends in Houston inquired if I was coming home for Thanksgiving. Undeniably I was looking forward for that as well. In fact, I mentally crossed off each passing day in a countdown to the holidays; but there was loads of work to finish before that. I was tired and the bed felt extra-soft and welcoming after the day's toil.

****

Consequences of Hatred

Never lose hope because if you
lose it, you will stop living

The autumn colours increased each day, painting the natural landscape with deeper and richer hues, proclaiming the rapid passage of time. My days were packed with classes and sessions with clients along with numerous other things that clamoured for attention. Time flew past so quickly that it seemed I was seeing my clients twice a week! It became challenging at times to remember by their names since many new faces had signed up recently. I remembered them better through their presenting problems, although some had sort of concerns. On Fridays, the sessions followed one after another and the day hurtled towards the last session, which was with Michele.

It was yet another Friday with the same routine. Rupa, my only persistent Indian client, who was scheduled right before Michele, was beginning to show some signs of progress in counselling. Now she had become more consistent about her concerns since the last three weeks. I guess she had started trusting therapy. Rupa was facing a hard time managing college and household chores simultaneously. Her husband who left early morning for work demanded the breakfast be ready early enough. Rupa having to complete her assignments slept late and felt extremely irritated to enter the kitchen early morning. This ongoing quarrel escalated to furious prolonged fights. Rupa complains feeling insecure as she scares her husband might leave her. Several doubts and fears filled her mind so ruinously that she could not rationalize her thoughts.

Rupa was progressing slowly by exploring her fears. My initial lack of interest towards her had now lessened, witnessing her genuine concerns. I took a few deep breaths and stretched myself a little after Rupa left. She often transferred her powerlessness to me, is what I often felt as we ended our sessions.

I was tired and still had my last client for the day. Michele was already waiting at the lobby. Michele was cheerful and upbeat on some days while on other days she was just the opposite. I never knew what to expect and each session was different from the previous one.

26 September, 2003

Session: 12

Today, Michele began as she settled in the chair, "Hi! This week I've been speculating a lot about my future, what would it be like, will I ever get married etc…etc? I feel insecure regarding my future." I was somewhat surprised by her direct urge to discuss about future.

"Michele, I'm wondering is there something specific which has forced you to think about the future, now at this point of time."

Michele nodded in approval. "Yes, I feel anxious at times and lately my sleep also has been affected. In fact, I'm still hanging in-between, waiting, waiting and waiting for Rachael. I've my fingers crossed! I want to believe, like you always say, that time changes for the better and it'll add meaningful chapters ahead. I mean—I'm productively engaged with school work, have an on-campus job, a place to live on my own, reasonably good friends and probably a soon-to-become partner, yet I feel hollow, incomplete inside."

"Well! In my opinion, you've come a long way since I first met you. Generally, the initial sessions for clients are the challenging ones, but with you the later sessions, where you unfolded all childhood memories, were the trying ones. You need to understand well why I'm referring to your past, I think that's the problem area and we need to talk more about it, so that you are able to see its unending effects on you. Once that's resolved, I see an optimistic Michele sitting in front of me."

She said, "I want to belong to the world you described the other day, but reality presents a different picture. Counselling has been one of the prime factors facilitating my strength."

"What else counts besides therapy?," I interrupted.

"Rachael's presence in my life, my chirpy little sister, Emily, and my passion for writing, they all count. I feel living alone has allowed me to introspect and discover aspects about myself a lot more."

Speaking her thoughts aloud Michele began, "You know, my life has ample shades of grey but I don't know how to convert them into white. My world of happiness does not include my parents, is this unusual? I feel peaceful living away from them."

I reassured her, "I understand your concern–but you don't have to blame yourself or feel guilty; maybe you will not mind their presence as much once you 'come out' to them."

"I want to run away from this reality of telling them. If I

acknowledge my situation to my parents and friends back home, I will be laughed at. It would only lower my self-esteem."

"Well, I was only exploring possibilities. It's entirely your call to decide when you want to 'come out' to your family, I respect that," I stated. "All other factors being constant, such as, your affinity towards same–sex relationships and the societal taboo attached to it, you'll have to be strong to face all situations optimistically. Never belittle yourself because of your sexual orientation."

"The future is scary, present is stressful; the past was painful— I have absolutely no place to hide, no place to be happy," she spoke dejectedly.

"The past has been quite unforgiving, but nothing keeps you from working towards a hopeful future."

"The future is uncertain, I fear every bit of it," she repeated, shrugging her shoulders. "Uncertainties are a part of life and we learn to carve our way, through them. Do you think just by dating the opposite sex, all problems would have been resolved?," I prodded her gently. Michele remained silent. "No, but at least one wouldn't have had to hide one's partner like I have to. Some parents I've known are pretty okay about such relationships, but not mine," she sighed and shrugged her shoulders.

Soon she realized it was five minutes past 4 pm and stood up. At the same time I got a call from another client, which left our wrap-up somewhat incomplete.

****

The dim lights in the restaurant that evening created the perfect ambience for a relaxing dinner, something I often enjoyed with friends during weekends. The weekend was more extravagant in the US than in India. Americans slaved all week to party out during weekends. It was as if people forgot all their stress during these two days.

After returning home I snuggled into my warm quilt and settled down for some light reading. It was quite late and Patty's family was out for its routine Friday-night movie. The night nestled quietly into the dark except for sporadic noises from the central heater.

As I flipped through the pages of a Boston daily, my eye caught an article headed, "Adapting to Innovation." The article talked about our preconceived notions and troubles in adapting forthrightly to changes. It made me think about my own journey, thus far, in this new environment. Surely it was an interesting read and I could relate it to my present life. Besides, I thought I was learning something new each day. New changes, new experiences, or situations enabled me to think innovatively and assimilate the new ideas into my own beliefs.

After I finished writing notes for Rupa, Beth, Amy and a few other clients, the following morning, I started for Michele.

Process notes: 12

Michele walked in today with the fear of loneliness. I reflected on her childhood history and thought that perhaps it was one of the prime reasons for her underlying insecurities. This session focussed more on the emotional than the factual aspects. Her non-verbal cues were sufficient to express her disliking towards her parents.

****

With the advent of October, the festive month, the shop-fronts were decorated and came alive with cartoon cut-outs and the like, although it was just the beginning of the month, preparations for Halloween were well underway. Halloween is an unusually interesting festival, where children as well as adults dress up in costumes to become their favourite scary characters from Disney or fairy-tale world. It was my first experience of this wonderful and colourful event. Angels, witches, demons, elves, fairy, Spiderman, and ghosts came alive! It was one day when adults could relive their childhood again. Of course, dressing up was not the only fun-factor; as with any festival, it would have been incomplete without sweets. Children dressed up for the occasion–some stumbling over their costumes and others trying to keep a head-dress in place--went around the neighbourhood, demanding, "trick or treat". They would get the candies and sweet treats especially made for Halloween. I think entire America feasted solely on sweets that night!! Not to be left out, I, too, dressed up as Thumbelina, one of my favourite Disney characters.

Amidst all the festivity, nature was busy stripping the vibrant autumnal colours from the trees. They stood stoically against the wind, tall and bare, as winter approached. I, sometimes, had strange thoughts walking past those trees—did they miss the leaves they had shed, like we humans missed our old friends and acquaintances?

My thoughts carried me back to many known faces. Some college acquaintances, I wouldn't call friends because I never spoke to them, but became familiar with their faces from seeing them almost everyday. There were so many inconsequential incidents which weren't so important then. Now as I refer back they were a source of treasure.

I remember knowing a girl, Zoi, with whom I waited for the college shuttle everyday. She was fun to talk and mostly lived in her own fantasy world, and loved watching Bollywood movies. Not just that, she often frequented me with her wish to become movie star. Zoi was absolutely awed by the glamourous lives the film stars enjoyed. She would tell of even marrying a rich handsome moive star and become famous. I mostly laughed away at her silly thoughts. Later she got transferred to Mumbai with her family. I did not have her contact, but I still think if she ever fulfilled her dream of marrying someone famous and so forth. My thoughts had transported me to an entirely different world.

****

The following week I could not have foreseen Michele's issues or anticipate her response on anything optimistic owing to her ongoing insecurities. It would not have surprised me if she came up with a new or some other urgent issue. I had been almost accustomed now dealing with weekly topics with many of my other clients. Initially it was frustrating not being able to concentrate solely on the presenting problems for which they initially signed up; it also became hard for me to keep track of such half-attended topics.

However, discussing this concern with Dr. Sparks changed my outlook. She advised me to allow clients follow their heart and conduct the sessions with spontaneity. Every week, every session, with every client I began expecting the unexpected. Their stories often made me feel guilty of growing up within a secure, relatively trouble-free environment.

As the week began, I was looking forward for a fresh start. It was pleasant outside, walking past the fall colour foliage, to the train-station. Usual like Monday mornings, I had regular supervision sessions with Dr. Sparks. She always encouraged me to explore more about my clients. It was sort of addictive, the more I indulged the deeper I unfolded facts about myself and my clients.

Beth followed the session after the supervision. Beth unlike the other sessions was on time for this one. She had wanted to open up about a lot of stuff ongoing in her life. I sensed there was some history of minor abuse during her childhood. However, she kept it unclear for me to comprehend the situation well.

We started the session right away by discussing her childhood experiences. Beth was in tears when she finally disclosed being subjected to physical abuse by her cousin brother. She went into the details of explaining some of the situations when it happened. It was painful for me to sit through the session.

After such an emotionally-draining session I felt quite sad for Beth. I processed mentally that her underlying problem of diet control and puking after enjoying a good meal were like forms of self-punishment. It seemed she silently despised herself for not being able to confront the abuser and passively giving in to his wishes.

My clients had become a prime part of my life. It was not just a learning internship process but I had begun to identify their problems as my own concerns. Their sorrows and joys directly affected my state of mind.

****

3 October, 2003

Session: 13

It was Friday, late afternoon, I waited for Michele over a cup of black hazelnut coffee. Outside weather was dull as usual with occasional sunlight filtering through the Venetian blinds. It was only past five and the waiting seemed longer than what the clock showed or maybe I was getting impatient. As the aroma of the coffee wafted up my nose, my mind travelled far off to my fond memories of India; however, the faint knock on the door jolted me back to the Counselling Centre.

As Michele entered I noticed her gait which worried me. Her dishevelled appearance told me she was unwell, either physically or mentally. The curls of her hair lay in a muddle over her forehead and shoulder blades, as if she had forgotten to brush them. Her face was pale, devoid of make-up and her lips were chapped. It was strange to see her without any eye make-up. She wore an ultra-faded and patched pair of jeans and a wrinkled moss-green jacket, whose sleeves were folded untidily. My eyes went to her right arm, which was wrapped in bandage. Was she the Michele I knew? In front of me was a pale girl who seemed to have survived a trauma.

Michele interrupted my racing thoughts as she mumbled, "The past week actually felt….like hell! I forced myself for today's session." Her voice clearly reflected dejection along with exhaustion.

I managed to get my words out, "If you didn't feel good enough you shouldn't have come. It's always understandable under unforeseen situations."

"No, I really needed to see you this week."

I glanced at her bandaged wrist.

"Now this bandage stuff is a long story—I wish you could face-read without me having to narrate it."

I empathized and stated, "Feel free to take your time."

"As much as I hate doing this, I want to share it with you and get it off my mind. Last weekend my Mom paid a surprise visit to my place. I had no idea about it until she actually arrived; maybe she was spying on me, I really don't know. She's on the verge of disowning me."

I listened in silence without disturbing her flow of thoughts.

"I was preparing supper with Rachael, when Mom knocked and Rachael answered the door. Mom hadn't met Rachael before so I introduced them."

"How did you introduce Rachael?"

"I introduced her as one of my close friends, which Mom believed readily. Interestingly, she would not have believed if I'd told her the truth. I knew that never in her wildest dreams would Mom imagine us as partners."

"So you succeeded in holding on to your secret."

"Yes, but it was short-lived," Michele exclaimed. "The following evening, the three of us decided to go out for dinner to North End to gorge on Italian food. All along the way Mom complained about almost everything that she could think of; she also asked Rachael a lot of questions about her course and so forth. The only thing she liked was the food, thank goodness for authentic cooks! It was while returning that the real drama started. Rachael, by mistake, spoke about her memories of coming to North End with her previous girlfriend. Oh boy!!! I didn't dare to look at Mom's face. As Rachael spoke, I felt my face burn as blood rushed to my cheeks. Mom remained quiet until we reached and then simply restrained Rachael from entering my apartment. It was absolutely disgusting and the weirdest behaviour she could portray."

"It must have been embarrassing for you," I added.

"Of course yes!" Michele continued, "Mom behaved deplorably with Rachael. She denounced same-sex relationships as immoral. It was humiliating and frustrating for both of us, especially when Mom was denouncing Rachael at my doorstep. Poor Rachael, she remained quiet although she started crying at the unkind words hurled at her. Probably she knew it was futile arguing with my Mom and soon left. Mom's behaviour has broken my heart into pieces."

"What was your reaction?," I inquired.

"Like I mentioned earlier, my bandage is a result of this long, story. I was furious and in no mood to tolerate her lectures any longer. I shouted way louder than my usual pitch to let Mom know about my disagreement to her views and slammed the bedroom door on her face. She kept calling my name while banging the door incessantly. Soon I was unaware of any voice; blood spilled all over my wrist, then on my hands, fingers, on the bedspread. It was too late–I had already cut my wrist out of anger and frustration."

A cold shiver ran down my spine and I swallowed twice before forcing out my words. I could not believe what she had said was for real. "I'm shocked. You certainly shouldn't have attempted such an act under any circumstance. Self-destructive behaviour is never a solution to any problem; it only makes one more vulnerable. I'm quite worried about you now."

"No, I'll not do it again, I assure you that much," she promised.

"I felt bad when I came back to my senses later, but at that moment I was blinded with anger. I couldn't think of a better way to punish Mom. I wanted her to cry, shout and feel helpless for making Rachael feel so miserable."

"Was it your Mom who took you to the Emergency Room?"

"I don't remember anything; probably, yes. When I came back to my senses, I was lying in the hospital bed surrounded by a few close friends and Mom. I never wished to see her face after returning to my senses. The one I wanted to see was missing! They informed me that Mom took help from next-door when she found me unconscious on the bed, to inform the college authorities and admit me in the Emergency Room at The Fenway Hospital. I was saved," Michele ended.

She remained quiet for a while.

Only as a precautionary note I reminded her, "I hope you understood the repercussions of such behaviour. No one else suffered more than you did."

Michele instantly corrected me, "I think my Mom did!! She got petrified with this incident. When she asked me the reason for such a drastic step, I wish I was bold enough to let her know that I too am very much a part of the community she despised; however, I chose to remain silent. She did not accept my reason and kept nagging for the truth, though I didn't disclose the truth."

Wishing her a speedy recovery I added, 'It's quite unnerving when parents act irrationally and are insensitive towards their children's emotional needs. The week has taken its toll on you very harshly indeed."

"Yes indeed! Finally Mom left yesterday and now my apartment is peaceful again. In retrospect, reviewing all that had happened the past week, I see one good thing emerge. I think the situation taught me to fight back, something I used to avoid earlier. Yes, I think I've learnt to become assertive somewhat."

"It's certainly good to stand up for your feelings, though this isn't the best way to do so. Self-harming acts are not worthy of any justification. Let this be the first and the last time," I voiced quite firmly to emphasise the seriousness of the matter.

My session with Michele today was a very different, something I had never faced before with anyone. I knew my supervision session with Dr Sparks would be immensely valuable in this regard. Envisioning myself as Michele's guardian now, I was not there just to help her with her mental tribulations; her act had made me apprehensive about her safety. Certainly this was not expected of Michele, a girl who shed tears at every session, got emotionally carried away and then to rebel in such an impulsive act. It was past 4:30, the Counselling Centre was closing down. I jotted the following before wrapping up for the day:

Process notes: 13

Michele indulged in self-destructive behaviour by cutting her wrist thrice. It was an impulsive act, she acknowledged, in response to her mother's offensive behaviour towards her girlfriend. I wondered if she had deliberately rolled up her sleeve to show that she was injured. She had already heard enough lectures so I did not want to reiterate those again. I felt sorry for Michele today. Her mother is unaware of the fact that Michele herself is sailing in the same boat and I wonder what her reaction would by if she knew.

More so, since she lives alone in an off-campus apartment, it becomes imperative to ascertain that she does not indulge in such acts further as a means of gaining control over others. Healthy strategies, like going for a walk or talking to a friend instead of brooding alone, might help. Surprisingly for the first time, I noticed Michele had no tears throughout the session. I wonder if this is the turning point; the girl who never affirmed her wishes now strides to revolt in the most unexpected manner!

I left the centre late that evening; probably the last one! The dusk had settled in its due course; the setting sun shone its amber rays on the trees, the brick-walled boundary of Simmons and other buildings. At the train-station, I vacillated between going home and the library. There were loads of assignments to work on and ideally, the library should have been my choice. Riverside, my stop for home, was the first stop from Fenway and it was hard to resist. So, I headed for home next. A thin layer of fog settled above the lush green patches on the sidewalks. It was the first mist of the season.

****

The subsequent week I spoke to Michele twice over the phone to ensure her mental well-being. My concern for her redefined our counsellor-client relationship and took it to the next level.

I discussed the incident with Dr Sparks the following Monday and she appreciated my initiative to call and keep in touch with her over the week. Also, during group supervision, Anne Marie, one of the interns, who had faced even worse situations of suicidal attempts with one of her clients, rendered a lot of support to me. Although this experience did scare me quite a lot, it also taught me to deal with such crises keeping in mind the safety interventions. In fact, the entire counselling unit provided me with much confidence, which further facilitated and encouraged me to handle the situation aptly.

It would not be wrong to admit that my clients helped me grow mentally; a truth I own with a lot of pride. It's not very often that one gets an opportunity to come across such varied diversities with a multitude of issues. I was fortunate to serve, which endowed me with a new world of understanding.

****

My Second Halloween

Acceptance brings contentment even
through the worst times

This was our 14th session; I was seeing Michele after a long gap of 15 days due to her injury and her effort to cope up with the academic course. Lately, due to her hospitalization she had missed quite a number of lectures. In between those days I frequently checked with her on the phone, as to how she felt. It was Michele who insisted on meeting for this session during our last telephonic conversation.

24 October, 2003

Session: 14

Michele walked in calm and poised, it seemed a lot more than two weeks since our last session. Dressed in a red, long-sleeved corduroy shirt with black pants, she looked pretty as ever with her hair pulled up neatly into a pony-tail. Initially, she was more reserved than her usual self.

Since she was quiet after the initial greeting, I urged, "It's good to see you this week; how are you doing?"

The bandage was still wound round her arm to remind her of

everything that had happened, Michele replied, "Definitely better than last two weeks. What I did was scary, it felt as if I was possessed or something. It was so not me!!"

Michele shrugged her shoulders and spread her arms wide open, as if questioning her own actions.

Amidst the periods of silence, she thanked me for checking upon her the entire time. "It truly felt very good. My own people didn't bother to call as much as you did, while I was recovering."

We both remained silent for some time. Finally she spoke, "In all the chaos that's being happening in my life, my most pressing concern is Rachael. I also called her and apologized on behalf of my Mom, but ever since then she hasn't reciprocated my call even once."

"Did she visit you at the hospital?," I inquired.

"No, in fact she wasn't even aware that I was admitted in the Emergency Room. It was through one of our mutual friends who informed her about me. She was horrified and got mad at me for such rash behaviour. Rachael consoled me that she'd never compromise on losing a special friend on such silly matters. I was delighted somewhat on hearing her thoughts."

I repeated, "Silly matters, ah-ha! So she actually mentioned your Mom's anger as a silly matter?"

Instead of responding agreeably, which I thought she would, Michele claimed, "Well yes! I thought so too, but after that she never called again. I don't know what's keeping her from calling me. I don't think distance would do us apart. Do you?" I was certainly not in a position to speak on behalf of Rachael and remained silent.

"I have thought about it, but don't want to make it too obvious that I'm missing her badly. Besides, I am a bit apprehensive about calling; what if she hangs up on me? After dealing with my Mom, I am not ready for yet another set of crises."

"I agree it's hard! Waiting period always seems longer than it is actually."

Immediately, Michele exclaimed, "You know, often I wish I was straight like everyone, maybe life would have been easier, like I always keep telling you."

I confronted her, this time a bit sternly, "Do you think sexual orientation is the only factor that causes complications?"

She smiled embarrassedly and admitted, "No, I think that was quite a lame statement. What I meant was being a lesbian is an addition to the already existing stress factors. I think of it like an added baggage to deal with. It's my loss if Rachael breaks our friendship I wouldn't blame her."

Lately, I've been thinking of registering myself for yoga or Art of Living classes to destress. What do you suggest?"

I immediately thought of encouraging her to join either, but that would have been more like a friend than a counsellor, so I restrained myself. Alternatively I suggested, "Let's explore a bit more on these thoughts. In fact, don't dwell on what others think about joining such classes, concentrate on your own views."

Michele seemed confused like always; although I was not blunt, she felt a bit intimidated. Nonetheless, she readily agreed. "That's right. It's more about me and not so much about what others suggest, but lately all my decisions have gone awry."

There was a momentary pause before she added, "Think I'll

get myself registered for the yoga classes, it might help my overall well-being."

"Now that you're looking forward to it, I would affirm it as an excellent idea. Yoga is a wonderful holistic approach and will uplift your mental well-being along with all its physical benefits," I concurred.

"Last night I couldn't sleep. I kept tossing and turning until some weird sound outside jolted me fully awake. While in my warm bed, I remembered the cold hospital cot, Mom's incessant sarcasm and her infuriated tirade against Rachael, the agitation that engulfed me and drove me to cut myself, the moment when Rachael walked away in tears. It seemed more frightening the second time, worse than a nightmare."

"Certainly I agree it is scary, but life goes on. Change happens for good, maybe this was an eye-opener for you. When you actually plan to confide in your mother, you'll be prepared then."

"It's undoubtedly scary ever since I witnessed Mom's rage, her views, her narrow-mindedness—I don't think I'll ever tell her."

"Mom's presence disturbs you, is that what you mean?," I asked. I deliberately repeated her so that Michele could get a perspective on what she had said. She was a bit hesitant at first, but she did establish that her mother disturbed her peace of mind, individuality, and confidence. "I feel crushed under her dominance."

As we were approaching the end of the session, I urged Michele to continue her thoughts in the forthcoming week. I watched her wordlessly step out at the end of the session.

After the session I did not feel like processing her notes. There was not anything too upsetting or disturbing that restrained me, but I did not have the inclination to write. It had been almost three months now, I was hopeful that Michele would emerge out of this vicious cycle of fear and self-blame; but often the sessions felt stagnant. There wasn't much progress, instead we were beating around the same problem again and again.

No one had said counselling would be easy or did I simply imagine it to be, I wondered. My clients meant a lot to me, just as improvement gave me impetus to trust in talk–therapy; their lack of growth weakened me.

****

The entire week went in a jiffy. Many of my appointments were cancelled as people were planning to travel over the long weekend. Michele too cancelled her session due to Halloween. Dr. Sparks was also out of station for a seminar, so I had an extra slot during the supervision hour. A day before Halloween I and Amanda ventured through the party city stores. It was fun watching the wide range of costumes. We even tried wearing a couple of them. Amanda bought herself a pair of fairy wings and I got butterfly head-gears for my self. It was a good break from my busy schedule.

Patty, Daniel and Shelby were home on Halloween night and enjoyed distributing candies and goodies to the neighbourhood children who were dressed as various interesting characters such as angels, witches, elves, ghosts, Batman and a host of other characters. The costumes, wings and the elaborate head-gear, adorned with feathers, nets, satin and beads, which people wore to mark the occasion were all made to perfection with exceptional detailing.

Last year on Halloween, I was at my aunt's place at Rochester, NY, with my family. It was my first festive event in the US. The "trick-or-treat", where children of all ages visited their neighbourhood in costumes to get goodies and candies was a custom followed mostly after sunset. The younger children were escorted by their parents for the occasion. My aunt had prepared home-made sweets specially to give out. All the front lawns of the houses were decorated with jack-o-lanterns and pumpkin shells with candles placed inside which glowed through the "faces" cut out on them, a speciality in Halloween; it was all so much fun.

I was celebrating my second Halloween at Patty's house because I could not get leave from my internship. I missed my family and friends in Houston, memories of the first Halloween kept coming to my mind sporadically though I did speak to them. I was not quite enjoying the candies and other goodies and found it an effort to even wear the head-gears, unlike the previous year. I spent the evening indoors, watching TV, chatting with Patty and Daniel as they shared their previous memorable Halloween experiences.

There were several Halloween parties around the neighbourhood. I was invited in two of them, but did not have the inclination of attending them. Amanda had gone with her boyfriend to a Halloween party which was arranged in a pub. A few of my friends from our internship had planned an outing for Sunday morning. I knew it would be lot of fun. We went out to watch a thriller movie and later stopped for an wholesome lunch at a Chinese restaurant.

Post-Halloween, the week ahead was a busy one with the approaching due-dates for submission of term-papers and the like. I was becoming more inclined towards seeing clients rather than writing papers. However, that was not a good enough excuse to neglect it either! The new week also brought the advent of a new month, November–the month of harvest and family reunions, colours and lights–the month of Thanksgiving. In spite of the pressure of work, I looked forward to it. But I missed Diwali back in India. Many significant memories related to the festival, which became ever so special now, made me more nostalgic.

Thanksgiving, a festival of harvest celebrated in the US, was equally as colourful. The month was significant for bonding with family, reunions, and dinner parties. Observed on the last Thursday of November, the festival gives plenty of excuses for shopping and partying all through the month! I was no exception to this and went on a shopping spree as well though more than that I waited eagerly for my vacation. I longed to be with my family; it seemed like rejuvenation for better performance.

****

The advent of the final semester caused Michele to miss a couple of more sessions. Although we met sporadically, the intensity of the connection between us increased. At the back of my mind I also thought of her absence, as well as absence of my other clients, as a pseudo practice before the final termination of their therapy.

7 November, 2003

Session: 15

I greeted her as she walked in smiling, "Good to see you, how are you doing?"

"Just hanging in there, tired basically with all the submissions and work pressure, you know," she replied through a brief smile, "Wish I could hide somewhere and go off to sleep undisturbed."

I probed, "Are you sure you want to continue the session since you feel so tired. Talking about emotional matters might drain you further."

She quickly changed her tone, "Oh no! I certainly want to continue, it's just that I feel worked up mentally."

I urged, "What is it exactly?"

She mentioned deliberating on the past incidents and the recurrent bitterness, "I can't seem to get over it."

I listened patiently.

Michele continued, "Mom is the most dominating and persuasive person I've known thus far. She manipulates my decisions through her convincing skills and like a fool I always give in."

I added, "You mean she blinded you to take decisions according to her choice, which you now regret."

Michele instantly took over, "As a child, I thought Mom was infallible and always abided by her 'rules', so to speak. In the course of time, I found her perceptions to be quite inconsistent from what I was taught in school and so forth; she has the most obnoxious and incongruent attitude."

"Michele, I always heard a lot about hatred and indifference that you share with your Mom, I wonder if love ever existed."

She starded at my face in astonishment, as if I had asked her to relocate to some other planet. "Love—you mean love from Mom? I would be surprised if she even remembers how to spell it. It's that one thing which remains untouched in our home. In all these years I saw Dad hugging Mom only once, which was years ago. They did not care much to show their affection between themselves nor towards us. It appeared Mom and Dad, both, tried hard to portray their power and strength; there was no time for such sappy stuff."

"What do you think of love, is it a worthless emotion?"

"Yes I was taught to believe that love is a waste of emotions," she interrupted my thoughts. "I remember Mom had hit me once for showering too much love on Emily. During my teens, Mom avoided discussing such topics and naturally I became comfortable hiding my thoughts and feelings from her. Dad paid no attention and Emily was too young. She often preached, 'the tougher you become the easier it'll be to tackle the world. Love is for the timid and silly. It only makes one vulnerable with endless tears. The sooner you girls understand this, the better it'll be for you." She then smiled drily and added, "It actually took me some good years before I learnt the art of diplomatically dodging such thoughts."

"I'm surprised that in spite of such rigid environment, you grew up to be quite open-minded and romantic, if I may say so, refuting all those beliefs. How did this happen? I mean, what made you emerge differently from your parents?"

"Honestly, I don't know it either; but I was sure about how much I disliked Mom's views and in no way did I want to mirror her image.

I think the older I grew and the more I realized, the further I detached myself from her. I fear we may never be able to bridge this gap: every day and night, at each moment, I recognize it growing more and more. As much as I regret her absence in my life, I feel sorry for Mom because she, too, is missing out on the closeness we could've shared."

I sympathetically attended to each and every word that Michele spoke. "Michele did you ever try to express your feelings to her?," I urged lightly.

"Oh no, I can't talk to Mom about all this. I prefer to remain unheard and suffer than confront. She won't understand. She's impossible!" Michele exclaimed shrugging her shoulders.

"It's true, that the more I pull myself away from home, I feel helpless, having no one to rely on. It's the same for Emily as well, though things haven't been as bad for her; being the youngest in the family."

"It must hurt," I stated.

I asked Michele to reflect on how she would expect her relationship with her parents to be, five years down the lane.

"I know, it might be a bit strange to think of such futuristic thoughts, but it'll clarify your own expectations and thoughts in the process of analyzing."

Sliding back in the chair, Michele yawned and responded, "May be some introspection is required on this, I'll try to think about it."

I knew she was simply being polite and the idea was not feasible to her. After Michele left I thought about her situation. I knew it was playing hard on her mind. On one hand Michele was on the verge of losing her parents because they did not love her unconditionally; while her own happiness depended much on the acceptance of relationships. Michele openly accepted the lack of love and affection within her family and the repression was to the extent that she was forbidden to show too much care even to her younger sister. In this session she took an assertive stand which did bring some difference to her life.

In the next session I thought of urging Michele to reflect a bit on the future and how she might perceive her relationship to be with her parents five years down the line. It was as if I witnessed the beginning of a sapling mature into a plant.

There was pending work left for other clients and a couple of paper work which I was urgently required to do.

Rupa had been regular with her sessions now. She had been lately concerned about her troubled relationship with her husband. Her constant fear of being rejected permeated through her feelings. I felt she needed to visit a family therapist along with her husband, where they could talk about their personal differences openly. On suggesting the idea, she adamantly refused it since her husband was not too much convinced about going to a counsellor for such issues. I was looking forward to having more sessions with her, to tap into her emotions deeper and let her gain better understanding about her insecurities.

It was quite late when I and Ann Marie left work, the last two left. Ann Marie was a warm caring and one of my closest friends at Simmons. We often boarded the train together whenever we could. She often reminded me of one of my college friends, who also remained calm and poised during stressful times. I always got the support I needed from Ann. Though she had a heavy accent, I did not have trouble identifying with her. The night was cold and dull and I did not enjoy the idea of walking down the street in the freezing cold to catch the train, but we had no choice either!

****

Acceptance Brings Happiness

Change is inevitable–even
nature abides by this rule

Being the end of November it had become quite cold and the warmth of the sun could hardly be felt. Most days I woke up to an overcast sky full of clouds floating to unknown destinations or to sudden spells of rain without warning. Bostonians took it sportingly and were always ready with rain-coats, umbrellas and light jackets, in case it got cold in the evening. I, too, learnt to dress up in layers and cater to the unpredictable conditions. It was the perfect weather for enjoying a cup of hot coffee with someone special.

Only a week was left for Thanksgiving and I was caught up with the excitement while participating in the merry-making that all Americans indulged in. There were smiling faces all around so much optimism in the air that it seemed nothing could go wrong. However, my internship and courses entangled me yet more around this time. Loaded with work, I had become lousy at time management and could hardly scoop out time for leisure activities.

On Friday nights and weekend I sometimes sneaked out with friends ignoring the work load behind. I paid for those fun outings by compromising with my sleep, and working until late hours. I don't know how fast each week ended. The time between Monday mornings and Friday evenings flew away.

This week I had my last session with Beth, because she was leaving for Ireland. She had managed a transfer there, along with a part-time job. Beth was excited and I was also happy that she'd be united with her family again.

This week Michele lit up the room with her enchanting smile and her sparkling blue eyes.

14 November, 2003

Session: 16

Michele was in a rush to blurt out her thoughts without wasting a minute, "Firstly, thanks for suggesting me to think about my future. I thought it to be really a neat exercise."

I eagerly expressed my interest to listen to her.

She continued, "Initially, it seemed bizarre to assume my existence as a separate entity from my family, but then that's reality! Frankly, I don't want my future to be lost like my childhood; it's too precious to lose."

I simply remarked, "Good!"

"Instead of cribbing about them, it's best to be away from my family. I wish Mom had accepted my choice without any fuss; what a miracle that would be!" I interrupted, "It sounds like your mother's approval means a lot to you. What would happen if she doesn't?"

"I'd lack emotional compliance."

"Do you want compliance because you are a lesbian or is it something else?"

Michele thought for a while and said, "Well, that's a tough one! I don't know honestly but I feel homosexuality causes mixed reactions among most, so it doesn't harm to have family support. However, I expect the least from mine. I mean, what good did I ever get from them anyway? The fact that they brought me into this world isn't reason enough to love them."

I observed her facial expression change into disgust and hatred, "Michele, I've never seen you in such rage. Is there something in particular that happened lately?"

"Nothing specific, just that last night I was thinking and thinking…about Mom and Dad and the consequences we suffered because of Dad's irresponsible behaviour."

After a momentary pause she revisited, "You know, Dad had other women to cater to his sexual needs. Sometimes, I wonder why my parents got married in the first place."

She sounded disturbed. Her eyes were beginning to moisten.

I put forth a strange question, "Did you ever wish you could choose your parents?"

Interestingly, she remained quiet, neither affirmed nor disagreed with my statement. Disagreeing would mean she accepted her parents the way they were, which was certainly not the case; while affirmation would signify the end of the last bit of hope of connection. It could have shattered her internally. Instead she said, "You know, I try to free myself from such thoughts, but they often haunt me and disturb me deeply. My childhood memories only add to the disappointment."

Silence filled the room for the next couple of minutes. She chose to keep quiet for sometimes and remarked, "It's funny— here I am, talking about all this, and a week later I am going to be joining them for Thanksgiving. I wish Simmons wasn't closed for Thanksgiving; I wouldn't have to go home. It's a punishment for me! I'd rather be loaded with work and assignments at school than spend days at home."

I added, "Going home seems to put a lot of pressure on you."

She agreed and said, "And the worst part is, I'll miss our sessions. I can handle things as long as Mom keeps her complaints and advice away from me. Otherwise, I fear, we might end up losing each other forever. Recounting the past incidents I have come to resent the sacrifices she forced upon me which were spiteful."

"I see lots of bitterness coming out."

Michele bluntly asked, "Is that unusual?"

"No, I just wanted you to know about it."

Almost immediately she responded, "Now that life is slowly coming back to normal, I don't want things to mess up again. I feel Thanksgiving is a mere formality and probably the last one with the family for me. Once I start working, next year, it'll be entirely up to me to choose whether to visit them or not. Oh! What a thought!! I'll be free like a bird."

"You seem to be anxious about the forthcoming gathering and that might be escalating such negative feelings," I reminded her.

"Frankly, I never thought like this before, maybe I am overreacting! Anyway, thanks for bringing it up, at least I'll be more aware and check myself while I visit them."

"Vent your feelings freely in sessions here instead of keeping them within. 'Let go' is the magic word to take away stress and lighten up. Also, if you prefer, we could chalk out some precautionary measures to help you while you are on vacation."

"That sounds like a good idea." Michele exclaimed with a slight hint of relief. There was not enough time to continue with the proposed measures, so we decided to follow up with them in the succeeding session. My afterthoughts on the session came effortlessly to my mind. I knew where the sessions were heading for and added a few pointers before winding up the whole thing.

Process Notes: 16

This was the first time perhaps, as much as I recall, when Michele explicitly accepted her individual existence as worthy, irrespective of her family or her partner. I knew she wanted her family's acceptance, in the long run, to sustain her lesbian identity.

Michele clearly expressed her bitterness and rage towards her parents, especially her father. She blames him for all the misfortune that she and her sister faced, owing to his extra-marital affairs. It was playing on her mind subconsciously since she was supposed to visit her parents shortly for Thanksgiving. Therapy undoubtedly had loosened those emotions which Michele had pushed away to the recesses of her mind, which now overflowed with all her repressed annoyance, pain, sorrow and hatred.

It was quite a different situation I was in, trying to achieve a delicate balance between being a therapist and a friend. I was growing professionally while fine-tuning my senses on a personal level.

In the coming week, we would be exploring some of the precautionary measures that might come handy to her in case she felt emotionally drained during the holidays.

Instead of heading to my place after I left the centre, I landed up at the library to pick up a few references for the family counselling lecture. I spent rest of the evening with Amanda and Teri. Lately, Amanda was having trouble with her boyfriend because she needed more space in her relationship. She exclaimed that he was too possessive which was suffocating their relationship. Me and Teri, being single, had little to contribute but were silent listeners to her complaints. Later, we had dinner at BC Cafeteria—a steaming bowl of noodle soup was just the perfect comfort food I needed to fight the cold.

It was quite late when I reached home, Patty was already in bed; the girls were busy on the phone and computer, their usual routine. Shelby was not yet home. I hopped upstairs making creaking noise on the wooden staircase. I was exhausted as usual. It seemed as if I was in a waiting room where I came to sleep and keep my belongings, as opposed to living there.

The night had silenced most of the sounds, even the girls downstairs kept the TV on mute; except for a few irregular hiccups from the radiator, which Patty had turned on high before hitting the sack.

The weekend permitted a bit of relaxation, though there were lots of piled-up things to be done, which I had been avoiding purposely over the week. They were mostly my daily chores such as laundry and grocery shopping. I also needed to pick up some over-the-counter generic headache medicines and calcium tablets from the pharmacy. At home I rearranged my book rack and walk-in closet. Besides there were assignments and research work to be completed which couldn't be overlooked.

Siesta on Sunday was a luxury that I could indulge in rarely. I woke up refreshed to attend my friend, Cathy's house-warming party. I wore a black dress along with silver hoops for the occasion. Patty offered to drop me at Cathy's place or a convenient location. But she did not have to do that because some of my other friends, who were also invited, picked me up on their way to the party. Cathy had recently moved to her new apartment from her old PG accommodation. Although, the houses and flats in Boston were small for the extravagant prices that the realtors charged, but this one was just perfect for two. She had done up the house in pastels, keeping it contemporary with a hint of old-world charm; and her grandmother's silverware and some antique lamps added to its beauty, which she displayed proudly. Cathy was Italian, married to an Indian, who was also an ex-student of Boston College. She was a great cook. The salad, pasta, grilled fish and the decadent, mouth-watering Tiramisu dessert, were all home made. Cathy had taken pains to present the food elegantly. I had a feast; it had been too long since I had eaten good home-cooked food! I did not fancy myself as a good cook! I thought of Ma's fish preparations, which she is famous for, and, of course, all my other favourites that she cooked for me.

The evening passed too quickly at Cathy's. It was past midnight when I reached Loveland Road. Everyone was asleep and I unlocked the entrance door with my own set of keys. Rasky was the only soul awake and greeted me with his soft 'meows'. I was too exhausted to think or plan anything for the next morning. I found it hard to keep my eyes open any longer and fell into bed.

The week went by as usual, hectic and swift. Many clients had already left for the holidays so the workload at the centre remained relatively low. The Friday before Thanksgiving was abuzz with shopping and partying. Even within the centre, the staff was busy planning their weekend dinner and inviting friends. The college looked quite deserted; only a few of us were working at the centre while most of the other departments were already closed for the day.

It would be two weeks after Thanksgiving, before I would see all my clients. I peeped out from my window and saw how the golden rays brightened the brick sidewalks, lawns, and the painted roof-tops. Generally in November, the sun was only a weak presence, as the temperature remained quite cold even during the day time.

I missed the winters in Delhi, which I associated with the smell of oranges and shelled peanuts and, of course, basking in the sun all day long. Today was the last working day before Thanksgiving and the festive mood took precedence over all matters.

****

21 November, 2003

Session: 17

I turned around hearing the sound of the door open as she walked in and greeted me warmly, "Nice weather; perfect for a picnic or something." The conversation turned to the previous session and I picked up from where we had left previously, regarding her mildly-depressed mood because of her impending visit home for Thanksgiving over the coming weekend. It seemed she was doing it forcibly.

Michele admitted her reluctance, "I do feel sort of disoriented this week, am not able to concentrate on anything."

"That needs to be explored."

"I mean, my thoughts have been bizarre and maybe it's from the fear and uneasiness regarding going home. It wasn't this way but lately I feel increasingly jittery," she explained.

When I asked her to specify what exactly she hated about the Thanksgiving event, Michele admitted readily, "I think it is less about Thanksgiving and more about facing my Mom again. I don't know what might happen, which is certainly out of my control. The closer the holidays are approaching, the more I want to avoid them."

I inquired about her earlier Thanksgiving memory to which Michele rolled her eyes as if it was not even worth mentioning.

"It wasn't anything great. It was two years ago. As usual, my uncles, aunts and cousins came over; we all dined together for the big meal. Mom admonished Emily and I, secretly, not to indulge in more than a single serving of pie. It was quite embarrassing, because my cousins overheard Mom mentioning my so-called inclination to overeat to my aunts and they made fun of me the whole time. It was actually a consequence of a previous Thanksgiving, when I had indulged a big helping of pumpkin pie followed by another generous piece of apple pie with fresh cream. Mom had accusingly screeched across the table in everyone's presence about my 'manly' appetite. I remember leaving the dinner table without finishing my much-desired pie. Ever since then she makes it a point to warn me before every

Thanksgiving dinner. I've promised myself never to indulge myself, at least in front of Mom again. I find it really very irritating to hear her repeat herself year after year. It is humiliating to be subjected to her comments and sarcasm about my appetite all the time."

"That's not a very encouraging thing to do, what your mother did," I empathised with her about her embarrassment, especially in front of the extended family.

Then Michele continued, "I wish this year could be special by celebrating Thanksgiving with Rachael, but she's leaving as well, to be with her family. Actually, Rachael is quite lucky because she has the support of her family even after she 'came out' to them. I'll miss her."

"By the way, how are things going on with her? I didn't hear you mentioning her lately," I inquired.

"Rachael had called some time ago and we spoke for a while, and that's when I came to know about her plans regarding Thanksgiving. Hopefully, she understands how much I regret about what had happened, but the closeness we shared before is missing. We spoke more like casual friends than partners. I'm glad she at least called."

"Give her some time; it's only a month since that incident. In fact, for any relationship to grow you need to be patient and ups and downs are a part of it. Since this is not a heterosexual relationship, there might be, on several occasions, unpleasantness from both sets of parents or other extended family members. Under those circumstances, it'll be entirely up to you and your partner to understand each other and act maturely. Also, isn't it better to be away from Rachael for the holidays on a friendly note, than being on the verge of breaking up, which was quite likely to happen after your mother left?"

"I agree that's true. I hadn't thought this optimistically yet."

The rest of the session we explored the possible precautionary measures that could help Michele.

"You don't have to adhere to each and every advice austerely, but do whatever seems feasible."

She nodded in her usual way, like I remembered her nodding the first time when I introduced myself.

"I don't say this will be easy, but try it. Whenever you feel like losing your temper, just count backwards. This is quite an old technique, you might have heard of it before. I'm sharing this from my personal experience and it might work for you as well. While concentrating on the numbers, often attention is drawn away from the topic of frustration or anger. It'll help to keep your emotions under control."

"I hope I'll remember this at that point of time", she laughed lightly. I agreed often such things slip out of the mind, especially when engrossed in arguments. She also reminded me that she was feeling less stressed by writing in her daily log, but feared someone would read her stuff because there would be a lot of people around for the occasion.

I agreed, "It is indeed very cathartic to write. Even those unconscious thoughts and feelings which we often miss out verbally, find expression through writing. I'm sure you have some provision for keeping it under lock and key in case you decide to write there."

"Well, things change over time; I haven't been to my place for quite long now. Maybe my room has been shifted, I don't know—it all depends on the environment–maybe I might be able to write in bits and pieces during late nights," she ended disgruntled.

"Writing is therapeutic for anger-management; it can really help you articulate and vent your feelings without letting anyone know."

Seeing her perplexed about the prospect of managing the situation with her mother, I shared about another client who was in a much worse situation than her. To conceal her identity, I referred to her as "X".

"Unlike you Michele, X cannot afford to live separately due to lack of funds and is forced to live with her family even though they are not on speaking terms. She is also undergoing similar adjustment problems regarding her sexual orientation, a prime cause for her family's offensive behaviour. Now, tell me, don't you feel your case is better since you have the choice to be away and visit them only for a short while?"

Michele patiently listened while I spoke; I assumed it had helped her somewhat, to realize that she, at least, had the freedom to live alone.

"Emily would be joining as well, so that's good. I'll have someone to talk to. Besides, like you mentioned writing and counting backwards might come in handy," she said on an optimistic note.

"Before you take leave, I want to introduce you to something called 'Systematic Desensitization' briefly. It is a technique used for treating anxiety problems— the person closes one's eyes and imagines the least anxiety-provoking situation and gradually thinks of the worst possible scenario. Instead of running away from those thoughts, they are encouraged to face it. It's quite nerve-racking to start with, but gradually they learn to face their anxieties within their imagination, which is then practised within real-life circumstances. Similarly, we could also do this activity in one of the sessions if you think it necessary."

"Yes, I think we can do that after I come back, sounds helpful!"

"I'll let you know how things went, when we meet post-Thanksgiving," she added and wished me Happy Thanksgiving, and I did the same to her. "Are you going home too?"

"I plan to! Thanks for asking," I said.

In the evening, while returning from the counselling centre, I felt slightly relieved since one phase of the semester had almost ended. This was also a kind of practice for closure, soon to come within a few months, that is, termination with my clients. I wanted to finish all my pending work before leaving for my vacation, including the client-related paper work. That night, I wrote three process notes for those whom I saw that morning. I wrote the following for Michele:

Process Notes: 17

Michele seemed a bit nervous about visiting her family for the holidays. I thought, almost instantly, of the contrast between our thoughts. While I was looking forward to going home and excitedly counting days to be with my family, Michele was filled with pessimism and felt it was a punishment which had to be endured. I imagined a bird making its way reluctantly towards the horizon in an overcast sky.

After I ended her notes, I contemplated on Michele's situation for some time while sitting at my desk for a while, before settling for the night. This was the first time that Michele would be going home since I started counselling her. She did not have good memories of the previous years, particularly the last two; I hoped this one would bring a ray of hope for healing of old wounds and the advent of renewal of relationships within her family.

Family meant a lot for me personally. I wished Michele would get a warm response from her folks and reciprocate the same feelings in our forthcoming sessions. Her love life had been unstable in the past couple of months and now there was added family stress.

Relationships are the core of human connections. Often times when my clients complained about their romantic relationship, I wondered if "true love" really existed or is it more about the extent to which one can compromise easily. In recent times, when there is less concern for emotions and more demand on being practical couples seldom consider compromising out of their way for love. Love an emotion that changes masks every so often. Those who make it together are the lucky ones to have found the true companion. However, taking love for granted is probably the biggest mistake one can make, which can ruin relationships.

I wondered if I would have reacted the same way had I been in a relationship. Stress seeps into every nook and corner of our lives, even love life!

****

Family Reunion

Life is never perfect; we discover happiness
amidst imperfection when we seek perfection

I was looking forward to the holidays. It had been long since I visited Houston. The Wednesday before Thanksgiving was our last working day and I was all set to fly the next morning and return the following Sunday.

It was truly the best time of the year; everyone seemed to be in their best mood and high spirits. The festival seemed to be an occasion when everything seemed to be on a large scale, be it shopping or partying. The stores, sidewalks, lawns of private houses as well as community centres, were beautifully embellished with artificial corn, pumpkins, red potatoes and turkey, of course, the prominent feature of the festival. Thanksgiving being a festival of harvesting and therefore food, it gave opportunity for people to meet family members, however far-flung, to get together for a special meal. It was also a time to set aside differences and rejoice or at least try.

At the same time I missed Delhi as well. It was mid-November, I imagined houses adorned with twinkling lights, candles, shops stacked with dry fruits and gifts for the much-awaited festival of lights, Diwali. I travelled back in time to the memories of celebrating the festival with fireworks, music, traditional sweets and other treats; my favourite part of Diwali was lighting candles on the porch. It had been quite some years since I indulged in these activities. Festivals are meant to be joyful, but for many they are a time of stress. Amidst all the happy faces I saw, I thought about my clients and wished that they were happy too.

Unlike other Wednesdays, I did not have to rush for sessions or classes early morning. I preferred an early morning because I got an entire day to spend with my family as a bonus. Patty was kind enough to offer me a lift to the train-station; from where I took the train all the way to the airport. My usual stops rushed by, but my destination was not Fenway, for a change. I liked travelling light, so luggage was not a problem and moreover going by train was cheaper than hiring a cab. I could not wait to be on my way home!

****

Home was a different world altogether, so different from my everyday life in Boston–my work, friends and clients! It rejuvenated me instantly. I felt as if I had been transformed into a different person. I certainly loved the freshness and the warm weather of Houston. The sun was a treasured treat to my skin after the unforgiving temperature of Boston. It was truly welcome!

Ma was overjoyed to see me and started to cry. It took her a while to get normal, while both of us tried to talk and laugh and cry, all at the same time! Baba was very excited too, I could see the expression on his face but he was not effusive as Ma. I guess it is just the way men are, great at hiding feelings. Later, I feasted on a sumptuous home-cooked meal—Ma's cooking is unparalleled–was the upper-most thought in my satiated mind.

We celebrated Thanksgiving with one of our very close American friends, who had invited us along with his own family. After spending some time with our friend, we went home to celebrate in our own way–the Indian way! Friends came over and we arranged for a potluck dinner; it was great fun to be back and catch up with everyone. A few of my friends could not make it, as they were out of town on work. The night slipped away too quickly like all cherished moments do.

In Houston, the weather was quite similar to the one in Delhi in November, it had not turned that cold so it was quite pleasant after sunset. Morning walks were not as pleasant and fun as Boston, as most people preferred hitting the gym than jogging around in the neighbourhood or parks. During the day, I chatted with Ma since she was also on vacation from work and caught up with all the news about the extended family. We also went out shopping and had great fun displaying our purchases to Baba. I pampered myself with lots of delicious Indian meals that Ma was only too pleased to feed me. Afternoon siestas were something that I indulged in more than I had expected. It was great being "busy" doing nothing. Occasionally, fleeting thoughts crossed my mind about my clients, especially Michele. I also thought about Patty and the way she had been managing life with her girls and Daniel; and how Dr Sparks might be celebrating her vacation with her grandchildren. I had known them only for a couple of months, but they seemed like family to me.

My vacation was short but crisp; I was saturated with freshness. The flight back to Boston seemed longer and lonelier. Responsibilities, which I had put on the backburner for the duration of my vacation, began to reemerge as my destination came closer. I reached back on a Sunday evening which was dull, gloomy and overcast. I boarded the train back to Patty's place. The journey on the same train, with the same stops, had felt so much merrier while I was going home!

The roads were wet and some puddles in the lowland areas made me presume that it had rained in the last couple of hours. I pulled out my light jacket, which I had kept handy just in case it got coldery and indeed it did!

Everything seemed boring after reaching Patty's house, though she greeted me quite warmly. I did not feel like doing even my regular routine chores and decided to meet Maria, a classmate of mine, for dinner outside that evening. It was a good way to get back to my usual schedule.

****

Monday arrived, heralding a new week, and all the celebrations were over. It was time for some serious business until Christmas. I was all set to rejoin work. The nip in the air indicated the severe winter months ahead, nonetheless, my morning walk felt extremely refreshing alongside the riverside.

The week proceeded and I wondered if I had actually gone on a vacation or was it a dream? Needless to mention there was plenty to do. Interestingly, I felt very comfortable returning to the counselling centre after the vacation, maybe because now the centre was a place with familiar people around.

Monday was my supervision day with Dr Sparks, and this time it was after really a long gap.

She was dressed in a beige jacket with a crisp white shirt and the same skirt she wore on the last working day before the Thanksgiving vacation. Not that it mattered much, but people did notice who repeated which dress, especially with so many women around, I suppose it was inevitable.

In the first few minutes, Dr Sparks and I spoke about the Thanksgiving weekend and I mentioned how refreshing it was to be with my family. She smiled and patiently listened to all that I had to say.

"You seem to be quite close to your family. I can see you are in that same state of mind as if still back in Houston."

"Yes, that's true. I miss them a lot here," I admitted, embarrassed. "I guess it'll take a while to settle again."

"So, now you know how some of the clients feel after coming to Simmons for the first time after leaving home."

I knew exactly what she meant and valued her insight. "I try to understand and be empathetic as much as possible, but often clients feel shy or hesitant in accepting their home sickness. They all want to show that they are happy being independent." I further continued, "In India, though I shouldn't be comparing, children do live with their parents and it isn't looked down upon or taken otherwise. I guess it's just the culture that makes or breaks our thoughts."

I felt she liked my openness and ability to compare without being biased. I clarified some of my queries regarding clients as well. I also informed Dr Sparks regarding Michele's visit to her family for Thanksgiving.

The week started again, it never felt I had actually gone to Houston for real. All through the week I saw clients, old ongoing ones and new first-timers. By now I felt like an old hand at handling new clients, while just a few months ago, some new clients made me feel quite nervous and unsure of my abilities as a professional.

Good news this week was Rupa's approval on consulting a marriage counsellor outside privately. We had been exploring over this past several sessions, now she was sort of aware that this would be one of the best ways to make her marriage work. She contemplated on convincing Ashish, her husband. He was unaware of all her mental leaps.

I was especially keen to see Michele and know more about her vacation this week. It was past 3 pm but there was no sign of Michele. I had no clue if she had decided to cancel the session. The tick-tock sound of the clock filled the room. At quarter past three, Michele walked in with an apologetic look on her face. Although the session was shortened, I was glad she had made it. She was bubbling with excitement, which made me sure that her vacation had gone well.

5 December, 2003

Session: 18

Michele started the conversation right away, "I am quite surprised myself that I'm saying this that Thanksgiving actually went quite well this year."

I smiled, sharing her excitement, wanting to inquire if it was a happy reunion. However, I restrained myself from initiating any topic and chose to listen what she wanted to share. The very next minute Michele exclaimed, "So, at last, Thanksgiving is over!"

I was relieved to see her smiling while she spoke, "Sure and maybe this was one of the better ones."

Michele promptly added, "You wouldn't believe what happened and how things changed drastically over the past week."

I exclaimed, "I'm assuming it's all for good!"

She chuckled at that, "Thank goodness for small mercies, no actually, for big mercies in my case! So, when I finally landed, like every year, my home was beautifully decked up with lights, flowers, pumpkin lanterns, and other stuff. I recognized some of the familiar voices bursting into laughter inside the living room. Mom hugged me warmly as I entered, that was my first shock! In fact, I was a bit taken aback by her display of affection, that, too, in public. Something's wrong, I thought to myself, but also felt great about her unexpected warm gesture."

I listened quietly without interrupting.

Michele's eyes sparkled as she took charge of the conversation, "It was like breaking our initial hesitation, you know! Dad like always was busy with his friends and drinks and shouted my name aloud, just to show that he was aware of my presence."

"What about Emily?," I interjected.

"Oh! Didn't I tell you about her?," she asked creasing her brows. "She joined later, just as we were settling down for the Thanksgiving dinner." She continued, "It was great to be with her after a long gap. I felt as if now I had someone real to be with; my cousins, aunts, uncles and my parents are way too superficial! Maybe it's just me, I don't know."

I listened conscientiously often nodding at her comments to indicate that I was attentive.

"Anyway, the dinner went well and the food was awesome and, not to forget, home cooked! A wonderful variation to the palate instead of the canned and frozen stuff on which I live now a days." She swallowed once and resumed, widening her blue eyes, "And you won't believe— I had an extra serving of my favourite apple pie, that too in front of Mom!"

"Now, that's truly great news, calls for a celebration! I am glad you did!"

"I'm surprised myself. Mom was sitting exactly opposite to me closely watching what I ate. She finally interrupted to inquire if I wanted some more pie, which completely blew me away. I was startled for a while. She sounded so normal, just like any other mom."

"There's more to it," she added excitedly, "Next evening we actually ended up discussing about a lot of stuff. Mom flipped through our old photo albums; me and Emily as toddlers, our favourite dolls, our birthday parties and so many other memories. It was nostalgic truly. This had never happened before; I persistently wondered what had instigated her to behave the way she did. I don't remember Mom being so affectionate, ever, especially towards me."

I agreed, "That is a drastic change according to what you had previously mentioned. Maybe time and your absence have mellowed her." Michele disagreed with me on that, "I'm not too sure on that one, but she did admit being worried when I was in hospital and all the embarrassment and pain I went through because of her. It sounded as if Mom was being a little contrite."

To clarify more, I repeated her thoughts aloud, "Does this seem like a new beginning? Mom confessing her wrongdoing and you also got to know her more closely."

Michele bent slightly forward, as if she wanted to confide something, "That's absolutely what I felt! I wanted to hug Mom right then and there and burst out into tears that have weighed me down since childhood, which I couldn't share with anyone, tears that longed for a warm touch. I wanted to share so much with Mom, but I didn't. It was like I had actually met my Mom for the first time."

Her nose was red and I sensed a lump in her throat after she had expressed those emotions. Though I was becoming attuned to Michele's inner sense of joy, I was forced to interrupt her in the middle of her thoughts due to lack of time.

"I want to hear more about this, but since we started late today it's almost time. Can we continue it in the subsequent session?"

Michele looked at me agreeably while I concluded, "It's indeed very encouraging to know about your recent developments. I hope this would be a very different weekend for you as well."

I stretched back my chair while feeling the vibrancy of the space after she left the room. My clients had nothing personal to do with me but I felt connected to them. They were not my friends for whom I missed or cried for but they were individual people for whom I felt responsible. I reiterated the session in my head. It was good that I let Michele initiate the conversation. This was something I learnt from my supervisor, Dr Sparks., who believed that clients naturally bring up an issue if it is important enough to be discussed.

This was certainly a significant transition in Michele's life. I was glad there were occasions when she felt close to her Mom especially while viewing their childhood snaps together.

She eased herself out on the chair and gently smiled seemingly relaxing from within. Her face and posture seemed less strained. Since I had known Michele for a while, I became reasonably accurate in identifying her facial expressions and moods. She left the room leaving behind an air filled with hope. In my heart I, too, felt optimistic about this new change. I simultaneously thought about Michele's discontinuing therapy. Was I insecure? I wanted to see my clients happy, then why did I feel this way?

****

The day faded into the evening gradually. Winters had settled in Boston now, and would prevail for the next several months to come. There was central heating inside each of the buildings to protect against the freezing temperatures, but the cold had to be endured when walking towards the train-station or the parking lot or even visiting the nearby grocer, for that matter. I thought it might snow; the first snow of the season and of my life but it did not.

I was not left with many choices, and headed to the library to use some resources for my forthcoming paper on group counselling. I was tired but who cared! Before leaving the library, I emailed Dr Sparks regarding my afterthoughts this evening. This is what I wrote:

"Dear Dr Sparks,

This is something which had been on my mind ever since I

finished the session with my last client for the day, Michele. I wanted to get some feedback from you regarding my feelings through email since you are out of town at present.

Michele had an unexpected but splendid experience of her parents during Thanksgiving. She is thrilled by her mother's affectionate gestures, which she had longed for from the time she was a child. All things said and done, the family had a great time. I was glad too! Michele has always been the deprived one, as you know, and this was just what she needed to reconnect with them. Things are working out just the way she had desired.

I know this is very selfish on my part to think, 'what if she terminates counselling?' Although I never want to withhold my clients in sessions just because of our therapeutic bonding, I do not know why I felt this way. This is the reason I am writing to you, could you please explain my undergoing insecurities?

All my sincere apologies for disturbing you during your time off, I hope you will be able to throw some light on my thoughts.

Have a great weekend ahead!

Sincerely, XXX"

Writing to Dr Sparks was therapeutic itself. Sometimes, our own experiences make more sense, much more than our bookish knowledge. I felt quite relieved after writing. It seemed just as Michele and other clients shared their tribulations with me, I shared mine with Dr Sparks.

****

Let it Snow, Let it Snow!

Hope brings an optimistic ray of light;
it makes life worth living

It was about 9 am I had just taken a nice warm shower and was getting ready to start writing one of my assignments, when I peeped out of the window and could not believe my eyes— it was happening—snowfall! In my excitement, I could hardly find anything warm to wear and without losing a moment simply leapt down the wooden stairs in whatever I was wearing, unbolted the front door and stepped out. It was as if I was transported to my dreamland. The light cottony snowflakes floated all around; they covered the tip of my nose first, then my fingers, the sleeves of my sweat-shirt. Snow fell on my shoulders and my feet. I was experiencing the first snowfall of my life! I heard Patty call out to me from inside to wear something warm, lest I should catch cold. I was living my moment. This was one reason, among many others, that had attracted me to seek admission in Boston College. I noticed that slowly the pavements, lawns, car roofs, and branches of the trees–everything was turning white. There was an unusual light all around which I thought was maybe due to the whiteness from the snow. Two neighbourhood kids also came out to play; they were well-protected from the cold unlike me. I watched them make snowballs and throw on each other. Their gloves were all white by the time they had made a few snowballs.

I wanted to do the same and play with snowballs. Being single was no fun, I had no warm hugs to give or to get in the freezing cold! After a while I began to feel the cold creep over me. My thighs felt numb inside the corduroy pyjamas and so did my bare fingers. I was freezing now and could not remain outside any longer.

Patty was amused to see my impulsive reaction to the snowfall. I glanced at the lobby mirror once I was inside and went back for a second look. My hair was all white by now! I remembered the song “My Favourite Things” from the movie “The Sound of Music”. I felt like Julie Andrews and sang softly, “Snowflakes that stay on my nose and eyelashes. Silver white winters that melt into spring; these are a few of my favourite things,” and climbed up the stairs without dusting off the snow from my hair or sleeves. I was thrilled and called up my friends in India especially to share my experience. Later throughout the day, it kept snowing sporadically. I heard puff-puff sounds on the wooden roof; it was different compared to the sound of loud rain.

Later, I went outside to run a few errands, it was wonderful how everything was covered in cold white; everything seemed so still and quiet. It was not that cold as I had expected it to be; rather the previous night was much colder. There were hug heaps on snow piled on the sidewalks, probably from shovelling the driveways. Nothing except the snowfall was new or worth mentioning that weekend.

On Sunday 4 at 6 am, I headed out for a stroll–it was nothing like I had seen or felt before. Boston was now transformed into a whole new world; my same old surroundings had changed from what it was during summer or autumn. I could feel the changing seasons so keenly, each one was alluring. The snow had its own charm and I loved it, except when it transformed into ice and started melting. There were more occasions than I can count when I slipped on ice, because it lay translucently on the roads. Luckily, I never had any serious injuries, but sometimes it did hurt very painfully.

Teri often grumbled about the weather being nasty every time it snowed. She was from Mexico, where the climate is similar to that of Houston or other southern parts of the US which do not have snow in winter. She found it hard to bear such weather conditions. Her looks were typical of her origin; she was a brunette with curly hair and dark brown eyes. However, it was her Hispanic accent that I loved when she spoke in English; she pronounced the "t" sounds softly, which made it sound exotic. Teri often invited me to visit Mexico, but during vacations I preferred going home more. "Maybe after we graduate, I'll come," it was my standard reply to which she smiled as if I was joking. Many thoughts lingered as I returned back after my morning walk through the snow, only few people actually went out for a walk during this time of the year. They avoided the snow and preferred working out at the gym but diehard lovers of snow like me could not be indoors!

Later during the day, I checked my email to see if Dr Sparks had replied. One thing I really appreciated about the people here were the prompt replies of all email queries. Dr. Sparks had replied my concern.

"Dear XXX,

I am glad you thought about sharing your concern with me. Please feel free to do so even when I am away on vacation, hearing from my interns is always a pleasure.

I understand your concern which is bothering you regarding Michele. On surface it seems somewhat selfish, as you might not want to 'let go' of her, but there might be other nuances to it.

Firstly, never feel sorry for feeling a specific way. All that we feel, think, or emote has an underlying legitimate reason, nothing is baseless. It is true that Michele has been among your most regular and favourite clients, but that is not the only reason you fear her termination. It is possible you are still unsure if she will be able to make the ends meet all by herself, emotionally that is. Sometimes terminations become hard simply due to this reason and as counsellors we get accustomed to know about our clients' well being. It is not unusual to feel anxious when losing that connection.

Second, I would like to mention, it is always good to be prepared for terminations mentally because clients are like clouds and they float away soon before one realizes. Michele might discontinue therapy; yes it is possible, nonetheless I am happy to know about her recent developments.

Accept your inner instincts and feelings as they will always prepare you to face the forthcoming situation better.

Keep me posted!

Dr A. Sparks."

It was indeed a well-thought decision to discuss my thoughts with her through email. I felt better and also somewhat confident about my feelings. Possibly, maybe Michele was thinking of discontinuing therapy and my instincts were right this time.

****

This week Michele was precisely on time for her session. I had been sitting with clients all day long, there were no missed appointments; and the staff meetings in between sapped all the energy out of us. All that we interns could do was just exchange glances as our supervisors kept on going with their usual routine.

She had been coming late since the last few sessions; I expected she would be for this one too. It actually would have been good because I was desperate for a short break in between my sessions. Contrary to my wishes, she walked in smiling as usual right on time.

12 December, 2003

Session: 19

Michele carried herself in a beautiful ethnic outfit; a reddish orange skirt with a white halter neck, which I noticed only after she took off her winter coat. I could not resist asking, "You look great but aren't you cold in that halter neck?"

Although I mostly desisted from commenting on my clients' attire, I could not resist this time. Also, I knew she would not feel offended, knowing her comfort level over all these past sessions.

There was a quick giggle, hearing my concern and she readily agreed, "Well, well! You are right, it is freezing outside and that's why I am wearing this extra-heavy snow coat and since it's quite comfy inside I am comfortable. Actually, I dressed up because I'm seeing Rachael tonight for dinner, and I'll be heading there, straight after this session." She smiled shyly.

"However, coming back to my Thanksgiving experience, this weekend I was home and reflected upon the relationship I share with Mom. I want to explore more on the recent changes I noticed in her attitude. I often feel time is flying ahead of me and before I can understand situations, they are over."

I reminded her, "Don't worry, soon it'll be time to visit them again." She was aware of the fact and responded, "Yes, I realize that. This time I won't fuss that much about going home!"

I also inquired about Emily's response to this entire situation.

"Emily too felt it was abnormal and unexpected to have Mom behave the way she did. I wish we weren't deprived of this affection while growing up, you know what I mean?"

"It's much like wanting a second childhood with Mom again," she continued.

Towards the end of the session Michele informed me of what Emily had shared with her. She said, "Emily's words made a lot of sense, although I was surprised! Recently owing to the unbearable clashes between them, my parents decided to see a marriage or family counsellor, whom my sister also visited twice, before leaving for college, with Mom and Dad."

This was something I always thought about but desisted, asking Michele as to why her parents had not sought professional help.

"What did you think of their decision?," I asked.

She was all praise about and spoke frankly, "There have been a million times when I thought of insisting that my parents consult a counsellor, but never had enough courage to say so explicitly. I was overjoyed when Emily told me about it; only if Mom had confided this to me herself, I would have felt she really valued my presence. Still, I'm happy about it!"

A few minutes past before Michele added, "Mom surely has exhibited dramatic transformations in her overall attitude, but I wonder how it has helped my Dad. He seemed to be the same old uncaring self!"

I assured Michele to keep faith and hope for the best. "Some incorporate changes gradually, while with some, it just clicks sooner. Needless to tell you, as you are a part of it yourself, that counselling is a process of discovering oneself, thus, it is a very delicate issue. Maybe your father needs more time to be receptive towards changes."

"I forgot to share something the other day during our previous session. Before leaving for Boston Mom actually hugged me, which I also reciprocated. I can't remember feeling like this ever before. It felt like I had been adopted by my real mother after been raised by my step-mom. This was the first time I felt a sense of belonging."

"There is absolutely nothing more valuable than the love and support of your family; and such emotional ties act as a source of strength during hardships as well," I added.

Her eyes filled with tears and her voice became husky. She further stated, "More interestingly, now when I'm alone or feel lonely, I just close my eyes and rethink of Mom's touch. It refreshes me magically."

Being unable to control my emotions I wept out of empathy. This was yet another moment of silence, of connection and bonding between us.

Michele was somewhat uncomfortable, I conjectured, to see me in tears, an experience she had not before.

She wiped her eyes and stated, "I'm fortunate to have a counsellor like you, sorry for making you feel tearful."

I reassured her immediately, "Well don't be! This is a part of the connection. I am crying because I truly feel your emotions."

Michele's blue eyes spoke while she remained quiet in the pauses during the conversation.

"I also want to thank you for being there for me whenever I needed support. I'm expecting this Christmas to be a memorable one. Santa has showered me with my most-awaited gift way before Christmas Eve," her voice once again cracked as she finished her sentence.

Besides family, I touched upon Rachael and her relationship with her, especially because she was planning to see her that night. I apologized to her for abruptly shifting the topics due to lack of time, which Michele understood agreeably.

"I'm glad you are meeting Rachael tonight. It'll lend you a chance to rekindle your relationship."

"It is a blessed day for me!" she accepted.

Pausing shortly, she continued, "I couldn't have been happier than I am today. Things are working more than my expectation. I wish Rachael would accompany me and meet my parents during Christmas, though that's too much to expect. I hope Rachael will be back in my life like before."

Those were the last thoughts we discussed in that session. Michele left the centre wearing her bright smile, as she did throughout that session as she zipped up her winter coat. I thought this was one of the most optimistic sessions with Michele after she left.

Sometimes it is a wonderful feeling to be a part of others' significant moments of life. I thank the divine powers for endowing me with such opportunities. It is true that clients seldom share their happy moments and experiences in counselling. In retrospect, I wonder, is positive reinforcement not as essential an ingredient as healing the negative is? I decided to write the process notes for her right then.

Process notes: 19

Michele, unlike many of my other clients, was excellent with expressions and words. This, in turn, enabled me to comprehend her thoughts and emotions more transparently. I empathized with her and wanted to hold her hand as a gesture of comfort, love and understanding, but restrained myself from any such actions. We were taught physical contact was unacceptable in counselling as it might be a gesture of invading a client's personal space. This was the first session where Michele spoke positively about her mother and probably, also, the first time she felt any connection with her. Michele reflected a lot more optimism than I had known her in the first session.

There was a sea of emotions, which I witnessed, while she laughed and cried simultaneously. It was obvious that she was excited and nervous at the same time towards restoring a new budding relationship with her family. Her relationship with her mother has undergone vast changes, for good, owing to her parents' visit to a family counsellor. I knew exactly how much she craved for affectionate motherly care. I am in no position to comment on Mrs Hobbes, but reflecting on what I have known of her, it seems she has been quite rigid in her approach towards life. Counselling might allow her a chance to relive and open up to more meaningful relationships.

Towards the end, we shared moments of bonding, when I wept with her on her account of narrated experiences. It only goes to show the strength of connection in a client-counsellor's relationship. In no way did I intend to intimidate her, or make her realize that it was too painful for me to withstand her narration. Deep within, I probably was missing my mother, which welled up as tears. A big milestone had been crossed during that session, not that crying made so much of a difference, but it was her underlying emotions, which I was able to gather well. I was learning to feel and to express emotions of my clients through my own body language, which was a huge stepping stone for me.

It felt challenging, exciting and hopeful after completing her process notes that evening. The session fortified me with a sense of contentment, or maybe it was the soon-to-happen closure. With each succeeding session, I knew we were approaching closure and that was not just for Michele, but for all my clients. I was preparing myself internally well ahead of time since my affinity with each one of them had grown over time.

****

Travelling back home, I squeezed myself inside the packed train, which was not that much fun. It was dark already and the weather was below freezing point. I had not expected the weather to change this drastically, so I did not have enough warm layers to ward off the cold. However, I did manage to reach my stop without feeling chilled since the train had the heaters on. It was fun watching the crowd–some were dressed immaculately with matching jackets, mittens and hat, while others tried innovative fashion. I always thought people looked cozy and more welcoming in the winter months by the way they dressed up.

The moment I stepped out of the train, it was like stepping into a freezing chamber. In only three to five seconds all the effect of the heating had vanished and I was feding really cold! I wished I had my car, or that there were rickshaws like the ones in India. My toes got numb gradually inside my boots. I walked as fast as I could through the sidewalks towards Loveland Road. The wintry beauty of nature was incomparable to anything I had seen before. It was like food for my eyes. The evergreens were mostly covered with white flakes, while other trees patterned along the street stood with their tall, bare snow-clad branches. They looked so neat from a distance, as if they were soldiers on parade. The driveways and sidewalks were piled with heaps of snow on both sides of the shovelled road. Everything looked picture perfect, but I missed having a companion who would walk with me. No wonder the weather was great, but I felt lonely at times. The quietness of the nature was perfect for a romantic night out. I waited for this time each day to walk and observe and enjoy the changes that nature wrought with each passing season.

****

My Best Christmas Gift

Nothing lasts forever;
cherish today before it fades into yesterday

The next one week, I was busy finishing backlog and preparing for the upcoming assignments and projects. The weekend raced by so quickly as if it were a fraction of a second and not days; returning to the same old routine of Monday-morning blues and the rest of the week with its unremitting workload. Where did those weekends go! Had they subsumed under the work pressure?

Christmas was round the corner, but who had the time to think of celebrations? There was so much work to be done before year-end holidays. Despite the preoccupations, the oncoming festivities pushed their way into the consciousness. The surroundings were already beginning to look festive with the typical red and white decorations; it seemed the entire US was engaged in hunting for the best possible Christmas gifts for their families and special people in their lives, while looking for the best possible Christmas bargains. I was excited because it was going to be my first White Christmas. I had seen it in movies and used to imagine how it actually would be; and now here I was all set to experience it myself.

As much as I loved the snow, sometimes I felt sad because all I could see all around me was dull blue and winter white. I was not used to seeing everything devoid of colour. I wished that I could share my new life, the snowfall, the experience of living in a 100-year-old cottage with everyone back in India. It is true we only realize the value of people when we are away or cannot visit them whenever we want. Only my thoughts could travel so far, while I remained in Boston. It seemed unreal how quickly we were well into December, which is also my birth month.

The Friday before the holidays I was required to submit some paper work to my supervisor regarding my clients. The morning started on a busy note–all interns took turns at the copying machine to get their papers printed and completed before submission. The latter part of the day was followed by meetings and respective sessions with clients. It was not exactly different from what the weekdays in general were, but since Christmas was around, everything seemed a bit extra-special or festive. The counselling centre had got into the festive spirit by putting up decorations. The entrance was done up with artificial red holly berries and leaves which gave it a Christmassy look. Tiny silver bells attached in between each of the notches on the door chimed every time someone walked in. Rene took a lot of interest and effort in all this decoration. It was remarkable how she managed a full-time job and yet had so much energy to expend in such special detailing.

One of my new clients presented me a box of chocolates as a Christmas gift. Since I was not accustomed to accepting gifts it felt a bit odd. Nevertheless, I thanked her for the thoughtful gesture.

Amy also gave me a greeting card wishing Merry Christmas. It was very sweet of her indeed. She had been under supervision of a diet specialist to check on her anorexic eating habits. We had come a long way I was expecting Amy would eventually come out of her constricted diet. We explored a whole lot on her past trauma and the hurt she felt. It was painful, but she showed a lot of courage to share it during the sessions.

****

My last client for the day, in fact for the year, was Michele. She had not turned up yet, although it was 15 minutes past four. This was unlike her. A few of my clients, including Michele, always gave prior information regarding their absence. I assumed that things were also busy at her end and that was why she probably missed out to inform. After twenty minutes Michele finally called at the centre's reception. Rene answered her call; I could only hear her say, "Okay, yes. Sure, I'll convey." I guessed it was for me as most of the interns had left and two were already in session with their respective clients. I heard Rene come towards my room, her heels clicking sharply on the hard wooden floor.

"Michele's loaded with course-work and sincerely apologized for not making it to the session this week," Rene calmly stated.

I thanked her and then lingered for a couple of minutes in my office before moving out. During those few minutes I heard the help-desk phone ring again. The call was transferred to my line–it was Michele calling. I was a bit surprised as she had already informed about not coming to the session.

19 December, 2003

Session: 20

Michele initiated the conversation, "Hi. This is Michele. I'm sorry for not being able to come today."

"That's not a problem. What made you call again?"

She hesitated a few seconds and said, "Actually I wanted to talk regarding going home. As you know next week is Christmas so I'll be going home. So—", her voice trailed away.

I took over, "I'm sure this time it'll be even better. Trust your own instincts and be yourself, now that you know things are improving. I will be waiting to hear from you when you return after the break."

She must have felt better, because her tone was calmer and sounded less anxious than the previous few minutes as she responded, "I am excited about going; it's just that I haven't visited them this frequently since I left for college. The previous visit was short and too good to be true. I hope this longer one would be as good!"

"Maybe frequent visits would make you feel less inhibited in their presence," I suggested.

She instantly agreed, "Maybe yes!"

I said, "Sometimes distance makes heart grow fonder but too much distance can even break the bond. It is good to communicate your feelings. With their change in attitude, maybe they'll accept you, irrespective of everything."

"Well! That's certainly too far a thought. I can't think of all that right now," she hurriedly stopped me. I knew Michele was unprepared to hear what I had just mentioned, but I still did it to check her response.

We wound up our telephonic session within the next couple of minutes. Michele thanked me, "I feel better after speaking to you." We exchanged Christmas wishes and she ended enthusiastically, "So, I'll see you in the new year the next time we meet!"

It felt good after the talk, simply because I assumed our conversation made some difference to the way Michele felt. I knew she needed to hear in affirmative to let her know that it was for good. Time changes and so do relationships and if it is for the better, then why not.

This was the first time any of my clients had proven me so right and reposed so much faith within me. A moment to remember my entire life!

It was the best Christmas gift I could have asked for. Truly, the process of therapy was so engrossing that often I forgot this was my internship; I instead felt responsible for all my clients' well-being. I suppose all interns felt the same. I had half an hour of free time after leaving the centre. What better way than to spend it with a friend!

Judith had recently moved to an apartment close to Simmons. End of a semester was reason enough to celebrate. She had been insisting since long that I visit her new home. I called her and we decided to meet that evening. I decided to walk to her apartment complex, only a couple of blocks away from Simmons. But I realized soon that it was not that good an idea. I should have taken a taxi or accepted her offer to pick me up. It was very cold and soon hailstones began hitting on my face, which was the only uncovered part of my body. I felt the cold chunks hit my trousers as I walked faster and faster. Very few pedestrians were on the street as most of them took shelter in the nearby local stores. As I crossed the red-bricked pavements on my way, I thought about my clients as I went past their dormitories and the Simmons College campus. A strange sadness struck me about termination. Soon I would be out of this centre forever and my connection with all my clients would also come to an end. I knew that my association was temporary from day one, still the attachment and bonding I had developed with them was not coloured by this aspect and was deep. Life would move on, so would we, leaving behind only memories of these counselling sessions. Unknowingly, I had developed an affinity towards the counselling centre as well and as days were rolling towards the end, I found it hard to accept that my time there would soon end.

The hailstones continued to pelt down while I was engrossed in my thoughts; soon I reached Judith's place, her warm and cosy apartment felt like paradise after the freezing and unforgiving hailstorm outside.

Judith was in her final year of school counselling; we had met at the library while stacking books. She was one of those people with whom I could share anything and everything. She was blonde, clear-skinned, and slim but still single. She often dated men but found them too nosy about her past life and ended up dumping them. She had her dog, Snoopy, who gave her a lot of affectionate company as only dogs can. He jumped around me, licking my boots and sniffing around, to welcome me as soon as I entered the flat, half-drenched from the sleet and hail.

Her new apartment was well furnished; I appreciated the detailing and the effort Judith had put in to make it look inviting. Being an artist, she did the walls with a couple of her own contemporary pieces, which looked very trendy. We enjoyed a wonderful dinner as we chatted about various things.

It must have been after 10 pm when I headed home, thankfully the train service was still on. It had started snowing and the night glowed softly with the whiteness from the snowflakes. Everything looked serene and dreamy; it was as though Santa was preparing his way in advance.

****

The following week, both Boston College and Simmons were closed for Christmas and the winter holidays. I went home for a very short visit but it was enjoyable. This was the best time of the year— to celebrate and reunite with family and friends; and to make new memories for life. I rekindled my old passion for baking during the holidays and experimented with cakes, cookies, and other baked items. The best and fun part, of course, was decorating the cup-cakes and the gingerbread-men with my younger cousins.

Christmas in the US was an experience quite different from that I had had till then. It was my second one and was even more amazing than the first. This time I got to see the best of both worlds–the White Christmas in the north and later during my holidays Christmas, Texan style, in Houston. It is hard to say which one I loved more. One captured me with its natural beauty while the other filled me up with the warmth and love of family.

The New Year marked a whole lot of new beginnings for many

of us who were graduating that year. While writing it was only a mere change of a digit, but the implication was far greater than just numbers. Many of my friends did not really care for the New Year, for them it was just a start of yet another year with the same old ongoing stuff; while some aspiring souls, including me, harboured new hopes and beginnings.

I was carried away by a multitude of emotions, both good and bad. The New Year indicated the final year of my Master's programme; it was an ending as well as a fresh beginning. With the new change I was sure to miss my routine at Simmons, my clients and all the responsibilities I endeavoured to shoulder, the crowded Fenway junction and a lot more other insignificant things which mattered to me.

The entire week went by so rapidly that I had no time to reflect or think about anything other than the work on hand. There was a lot—clients, case histories, meetings, the presentation at Boston College, submissions— everything piled up on top of one another. I felt unable to cope at times and wished I could just run away from all this pressure. The load kept on increasing pushing us to our limits.

Teri and Amanda too felt similarly. Amanda hardly found time to spend with her boyfriend due to which they often ended up quarrelling. "Managing love life along with internship and Masters was no joke," Amanda often stated. I and Teri laughed at her silly expressions. Though times were hectic sharing with friends made things easier.

I got a rude shock when one of my clients, who had refused to divulge any personal information, later complained to the supervisor that she was not attended to properly during the session. However, thanks to the wonderful understanding I shared with Dr. Sparks, things did not go out of hand. She knew I was undergoing a tough time with that client because I had already informed her about her attitude. It all ended all well when Dr Sparks and I actually sat with Cathy, my tough client, to sort out the issue. It became clear that she had been through bitter experiences with her previous counsellor, thus reluctance to open up became her natural tendency. Many a time, counselling amazed me with its spontaneity to identify the root cause of the problem. It has never failed to surprise me till date!

****

Towards Optimism

Relationships fortified with love last
through the worst test of time

I was seeing Michele today after a long well-deserved break of almost two weeks. I knew there would be lots to listen and lots to reflect upon.

9 January, 2004

Session: 21

We warmly greeted each other "Happy New Year" at the start of the session. Michele looked fresh and confident in her black outfit. Each session I saw her, she looked different from the previous session in terms of her outfit, and make-up or hairdo. Today, Michele's make-up took the centrestage. Normally, wearing make-up during the day would look odd, but she did it so tastefully that I never thought of her as overdressed.

She quickly picked up the conversation, "So good to see you in the beginning of yet another New Year. Now we can say we've known each other for almost one year."

I smiled and she chuckled.

"How was Christmas?," I asked.

"Actually pretty good, really needed a break from that endless course work; but now I'm back to my usual schedule."

When I inquired about her experience, she seemed even more enthusiastic than before, "I couldn't have wished for more. It was really good and the four of us actually sat together after dinner and lunch after such a long time. It conferred an amazing sense of completeness, which I have never had before."

I was happy that she found satisfaction spending time with her folks. "That's great, glad that things went even better than expected."

She nodded and continued, "You won't believe Mom has become a totally different person. She talks without any sarcastic comments. There's an astounding decrease in Mom's overall anger. Things at which she got upset previously, now she deals with them more sensibly, with tolerable arguments. Boy! I want to see that family therapist, what an outstanding job!"

"Your mother has truly benefited from therapy it seems! How does she see her change?," I probed.

It took Michele some time to reply. "Mom clearly admits that counselling has been a blessing in disguise, indeed for saving our home and her marriage." She continued, "The way I felt these few days is a feeling I can't really recall having felt in the last many years. Emily is also very excited about Mom's new 'avatar'." She said the last word with a wide smile adding, "Hope I used my Hindi skills correctly!"

"Of course you did! That's very impressive." I added, "How about your Dad?"

"He is still a bit arrogant and rude but I'm hopeful he'll change. I think what you had once mentioned that everyone reacts differently: a week for some, can take months for others."

"I hear some very optimistic thoughts, which makes me very proud of you Michele!" I exclaimed and furthered the conversation. "The first step towards change is acceptance, if one can accept their shortcomings then transformation occurs naturally as a byproduct of the realization."

Michele switched topics thereafter. She wanted to talk about Rachael which I readily encouraged.

She murmured softly, so soft that I had to bend forward towards her to hear what she said.

"I don't know and I never even thought I would say this, but I'm thinking of telling Mom about my relationship."

I was momentarily struck by her comment.

"What an optimistic thought! What made you think in this direction?," I urged instead of bombarding her with questions that were sprouting inside my mind.

She seemed firm yet doubtful about it, "Honestly, I don't know myself. I don't know what tempted me to discuss this with you. I haven't even shared this thought aloud with myself yet. This is perhaps the first time I heard myself saying this! It's sort of a feeling that's been on my mind past few days and just thought of sharing it with you."

I initiated a little push to endow her with the support that she was on the right track.

"You are certainly in the right direction. Don't lose hope and belief in yourself. The struggle might get tougher, but it's your own unconditional trust to win over your parents. The right time to disclose is when you feel it is right intrinsically; even thinking about this is a major step in itself."

"I feel," she began, "scared of Mom to confide in her, don't really care much about Dad. He might not even care that his daughter is a lesbian. Although I'm thinking of telling her, it is extremely daunting. I am quite certain Mom would get the shock of her life to know her daughter is a homosexual. Maybe she'll abandon me forever."

"It's natural that you fear losing her love, something you longed for so many years. Is that one of the reasons that you fear confiding in her?," I questioned.

"I won't disagree to that. It's true I do fear losing her love once again," she admitted, nodding her head.

"I fear the consequences and what life would offer once I unveil all this," she stated anxiously.

"Maybe you could give it some more time and communicate with your mother and strengthen your relationship before pouring your heart out."

She consented readily, "Sounds feasible. I was only discussing the pros and cons, but sure it'll be some time before I can actually disclose the truth." I put forth eagerly, "Thinking aloud would allow you to understand more clearly." She silently attended while I spoke. "The more you explore, the less anxious you will feel about the situation."

"It boosts my confidence when I talk in sessions without being judged, and maybe that's the reason counselling is different!"

I continued reflecting on her words for some time after the

session, until the phone rang, which was from another client wanting to reschedule her time slot. Before attending to the pending work at hand, I contemplated on today's session. It was interesting how things had shaped in her life. I felt good about witnessing Michele's transition in the past few months.

Michele was quite forthcoming in her thoughts this evening; especially about her desire to disclose her sexual orientation to her mother. Her Mom's positive attitude had bridged their communication gap to some extent and Michele wishes to further work on it. She is not sure about her father though, he came across as the same old person. Michele seemed quite well and relaxed after the holidays, which was reflected in her demeanour. The girl, who never even dreamt of "coming out" to her friends, was now ready to disclose it to the one person she feared the most, her mother. I felt proud of her inner strength.

Over the course of time, there has been a drastic shift in her realization of self-worth. It might have been a result of prolonged positive feedback in counselling and partly her mother's welcoming gesture of love.

Deep within I hoped Michele to never deny her happiness under any compulsions. I had no idea whether her parents would accept her sexual orientation, but anticipated that she would stand for it without being ashamed or embarrassed. All I wanted counselling to do for her was to make her realize her own strength as a woman, as a lesbian, and never feel inferior or self-conscious.

By the time I was done, the centre was almost deserted and most of the interns had left. Due to my evening classes I preferred seeing clients till late to utilize the time in between. Lesley, another intern, also finished her scheduled clients by then.

We crossed the lane and hopped on to the sidewalk to reach the Fenway train-station. The snow had been shovelled well across the streets so I did not slip with my high-heel boots.

Lesley was an African American though her accent was more like Americans. She had lived in Boston since her childhood. She was a single parent with a small baby girl. After working for a couple of years at a hospital, Lesley had decided to rejoin school to complete her Masters. It would fetch her better job opportunities.

We parted at the train-station. Lesley took a shuttle bus, while I waited for the train. On my way back, the train was packed with passengers as it was the peak hour, 6 pm, from the Fenway train-station. I never expected to get a seat, but if I ever managed one, it was my lucky day!

The winter had started testing our tolerance already. The combination of freezing winds with latent rays from the setting sun whispering underneath the clouds was simply spectacular. I experienced how it was sunny yet freezing! Nature mesmerized me with new surprises everyday; none of them were replications of the previous day. It was like a painter at work showing off his talent. However, for those who lived in Boston for years, or were born there didn't bother much about such changes. One person I knew among them was Patty. However, all this was new to me and I loved noticing every little change that really wasn't even worth noticing for many.

Weeks passed so quickly that it became hard to manage stuff, I staggered my schedule accordingly. During this time of the semester I felt the pressure was more than I could handle. I had no choice but to devote more time on my course work and papers, though clients were way more indulging to work with. Despite the workload every bit of appreciation from my professor at BC made my efforts worthwhile. I wanted to excel and do even better, they encouraged me and I pushed myself to excel until I was satisfied with the quality of my work.

The second week of January was quite sluggish at Simmons in terms of clients, mostly because of the approaching exams. Clients cancelled or requested for postponing the session to a later date. Seven clients had cancelled that week; it was the maximum number of "no-show" throughout my entire internship.

During the staff meetings and discussions with other interns, I found they were also facing a similar situation. I thought, "At least it's not me doing something wrong, it is truly the semester work pressure." Working with many interns always helped because it added support in exchanging ideas about the various issues.

This week I did not expect, but Michele turned up for her session. It was surprising because I knew she was lagging behind in her course work.

16 January, 2004

Session: 22

In the past 20 minutes we had been discussing about Michele's slow-paced love life. While she spoke I repeatedly heard her mention Rachael's confidence as one of the most enduring characteristics.

I softly planted a question to see her reaction, "How would you rate yourself in terms of confidence?"

"No one has ever asked me about my confidence," she

said reluctantly. "Initially I thought confidence was alien to me, something that didn't belong to me, maybe because I am a lesbian, I don't know!"

She carried on in a rather sarcastic tone, "No one cares about such trivial issues like Michele's confidence. What a big joke! All the confidence I have, today, is because I have taught myself things that maybe my parents should have. I think I've earned my confidence so it's even harder for me to judge myself. When I see other lesbians like me, living confidently and independently, it makes me feel optimistic and I am reassured that I, too, can be like them."

I probed, "Why do you think your sexual orientation might work against your confidence?"

Michele contemplated over my question, maybe she had not attempted to think this precisely. "Of course, that's for sure. Whenever, though seldom, I felt confident or praiseworthy it was mostly due to my hard work in academics and had nothing to do with my sexual identity. As far as being a lesbian is concerned, I don't think it'll ever make me feel worthy, it's just something I am happy to be."

I stated, while contemplating on these thoughts, "Maybe while growing up your parents projected such feelings on you, which might have contributed to insecure feelings."

Michele shrugged her shoulders, "Maybe! Growing up I felt Mom was quite irrational about trivial issues as such, people of colour, or lower economic status. Sometimes I felt embarrassed seeing her behaviour with our neighbours, she spoke only with those who belonged to a certain class. Most of my friends weren't that well-off because of which Mom seldom behaved well with them when they visited us. Towards the end of my schooling, I stopped inviting my friends home because I felt embarrassed."

"Precisely–that's what you too have started valuing–the visible academic success," I remarked.

She looked perplexed. "You are right; I do think my performance is directly related to my own evaluation. I remember Mom always detested people from minority groups and now I'm very much a part of it myself. How can I feel good about myself?"

"Your sexual orientation is only a part of you and not a separate entity by itself. Being confident or feeling worthy of self has to come from within."

"I'm learning to let go of my inhibitions and now after being in therapy for so long, I've started noticing subtle changes, like buying clothes of my choice and not of Rachael's to make her happy, something I would have done otherwise."

Summing up I firmly stated, "Well Michele you've come a long way! I think you already realize that life isn't a bed of roses and we all go through our share of sorrows. You have struggled a lot, now maybe it's time you start living your life in your own terms. Sexual orientation, in most cases, is taken for granted. People will always have different opinions, but you have to think progressively. You have all the freedom to choose who your life partner and if that happens to be a woman accept it with pride."

"A single negative remark can ruin it all", she said and narrated one such experience. "It happened when Rachael and I were at the mall walking hand in hand, a bunch of girls commented as they crossed us. It was hurtful, I don't exactly remember, but it was something sarcastic like, 'look at the love birds, poor things they couldn't find guys to hold hands with.' The other commented, 'going around with guys is old-fashioned,' at which they all laughed and sniggered. I felt conscious and Rachael got quite angry at their comments, but we didn't reply back."

"It's certainly very disappointing that there still exists such meanness in our society. I thought people don't really care in the US, but it's all the same globally; only there's a difference in the intensity of remarks. In India, of course, the situation is worse because people don't even entertain such issues as being worthy of discussion, some even think it's a sin to be homosexual."

Michele added, "I feel bad for those who are in my situation there in India. Well, it really helps to have a foreign counsellor. I get to know more about other parts of the world as well."

At some point of time I realized our conversation had begun to sound friendlier than professional, as we were discussing general concerns, attitudes and the differences between people in India and the US.

Over time, I had grown quite comfortable with some of my clients and Michele was one of them. We had reached a stage in therapy where not only did she discuss everything at ease, but also freely confronted any of my incongruent suggestions. This transparency was something I had not achieved with many clients; it was a reward for me, but I had to handle it delicately while maintaining the professional balance.

We ended the session on a lighter note conversing on more global than personal perspectives.

Later that night after returning home, when I conceptualized

Michele's case, it struck me the ease with which she accepted my confrontations. Her words clearly indicated lack of self-respect. It is possible that because Michele's parents never valued her for the person she was and constantly compared her academic achievements with that of Emily's, Michele learned to attach more importance to such gains than intrinsic worth. She needed to step out of her cocoon and rebuild herself, who would feel worthy of her identity as well.

I always felt very disheartened when my clients belittled themselves without reason. Today was one of those moments. I wished she accepted that attraction towards the same sex is not shameful, but a natural phenomenon over which she had no control, just as she had no control over being born to an Italian family.

I knew Michele was moving forward but at every stage there were grave chances of her regressing back to the earlier one. A slight push, I considered, was necessary to usher her in the right direction. I had been observing Michele quite vigilantly over the weeks and now, along with counselling, there were other positive changes like her relationship with her mother, to help her think optimistically. It was perhaps the right time for her to step out and face everyone confidently.

****

A New Reflection in the Mirror

We can be our own best friend;
no one knows us better than ourselves

Three back-to-back cancellations on Friday allowed me to redeem those slots for all my pending work. A couple of unfinished client reports, two reflection papers on family counselling occupied my time completely. It was about 1 when I had started working and it was 3 by the time I finished. Some days, like that Friday, were meant for theoretical work. I felt relieved after finishing it; it was as if I were decluttering my mind along with my "in-tray".

Rupa this week was late for her session. She walked in weeping and her facial expressions informed me about her distress. During the session she complained that Ashish was strictly against any kind of professional help. She had lost most of her hope of patching up her marital conditions. I sat through her agony as she shared the details of their bitter conversations. Undoubtedly, it would be some time until she could overcome the situation. She openly abused her husband for being so rude to her and left feeling better after venting out her anger. I let her speak her mind. "It's cathartic to be able to say whatever without being judged," she exclaimed.

Post-session I reminded myself that this was the same client who initially was so skeptical about counselling and now she was relying her marital peace on therapy. How out of the ordinary it was!

Michele was up next. She arrived at her usual time, 4. I appreciated her punctuality and wondered secretly if I would have been that punctual if I were a client!

23 January, 2004

Session: 23

It took me only a glance to notice that she looked different, which I addressed instantly.

"I do?," Michele responded, raising her eyebrows, "Yeah I was bored with my old look, so did some experimenting. I love my new look. It's really cool and happening! Rachael found me looking hot and after a long gap we made passionate love to celebrate our closeness."

"It seems like you both are back together for good!"

"I hope so too," Michele responded expectantly.

Michele stated, "One thing for which I want to thank you is the faith your have in me. You've constantly supported me to question my own irrational thoughts and behaviour."

I thanked her, "You don't have to speak words in my praise; I can already see confidence sparkling in your eyes."

It was quite certain that Michele was trying to and learning to change herself to become more balanced. I added intentionally, "Sometimes our body language speaks more than words can. I like your optimism today."

Michele interrupted, "I'd agree to that! Expressions and feelings can be articulated in any form and like you suggested, I've even started attending to my intuition without bothering about what others might think. Our last session actually shook me when I realized that self-confidence, self-image and self-worth are petals of the same flower."

What a wonderful way to express, I thought. She should have been a student of literature! I heard her voice continue, "Being a lesbian must not come in my way of feeling a worthy person. You know I especially got my hair coloured because I wanted to see what would happen if I go with my gut feeling. It actually worked!! Though my friends did appreciate my new look, but the most appreciation I got was from myself, because I could follow my heart and this made me feel very proud."

I affirmed her thoughts as encouraging. Urging a bit further I said, "I see you have acquired enough confidence and courage to stand up for your priorities in life. Today, if people are appreciating your looks, doesn't necessarily mean they would be as appreciative of all your thoughts. The real test would be to continue believing in your self without being influenced by their opinions, even when things aren't so good with others." She admitted feeling vulnerable to follow her heart when her thoughts were incongruent to others. "I feel very weak when someone gives me a nasty, inferior look as if I have committed some crime by choosing a woman partner."

"That's exactly my point, you have to be firm and let go of such weakness. Take little steps towards fulfilling your desires and when the time comes, I'm certain you'll be able to stand for your identity as well, irrespective of others."

Although she was expressive most of the time, there were instances when Michele remained silent and absorbed all that I said like a sponge. I presume she was in that state at the point in the session.

"You have to make a conscious effort to move out of this feeling of uncertainty. Recognize your inner strength before facing the outside world and it's something which only you can do. Though we all have manifold roles as a partner, daughter, mother, or a friend, our first recognition is who we are as a person, separate from all the other roles that we play. Never belittle your own choices, instead cherish them. None of us are born with high self-esteem or confidence; it is something we acquire through positive experiences, interactions and encouragement and all these endeavour jointly to attain worthy feelings. I know you have been deprived during childhood, but don't let your past ruin your present or future."

"I agree but one has to have that proper exposure and experiences to prove one-self. Second, one must possess the art of convincing others to their own benefit, which I certainly do not have. My Mom is an example. I mean, she can convert wrong into right just to boost her self-esteem," she said in a sarcastic tone.

"Yes, it largely depends on one's personality but even then you can exercise some effort at least to make yourself heard. Trust me you can!"

She quickly interrupted, "How to start?"

Within a fraction of a second I responded, "Start right now. You may even read articles related to how to boost self-esteem. Also take small steps, like 'come out' within friends about your sexual orientation, learn to take it in your stride if their reaction is not supportive. Besides, you can always attend and take proactive part in LGBT meetings. The more pragmatically you deal with it, the less intense it'll be."

She added, "Rachael really has come a long way, she accepts her identity in public very casually. I learn from her and she's indeed a big support."

As usual, during the last couple of minutes, Michele touched upon a relatively new topic. "Besides feeling awkward about accepting my identity in public, I feel concerned about having babies."

She further carried on, "I adore kids and want my own at some point of time. Adoption or artificial insemination are the options, but I don't know, it's all too early to think."

So, I simply repeated her last words, "It's really early I agree, but there's something which is prompting you to think about it."

"Well! I…I don't know maybe I miss my childhood and long to play with my living dolls, or maybe it's Rachael."

"What about Rachael?"

"Her commitment for a long-term relationship, I really don't know if it's at all related."

I shared my insight with her, "I may be wrong, but it seems you are thinking about babies, while unconsciously it's actually assurance and commitment that you are looking for."

Michele was unexpectedly surprised by the feedback I gave.

She cried out, "Goodness gracious! I would have never thought this way, you know. Certainly you got me thinking, is this abnormal or what?"

"No not at all! Nothing is abnormal; in fact what is normal for one may not be so for the other. It's not as daunting as you think. It's quite natural to undergo such insecurities when we expect more from our loved ones."

She urged, "Yeah, right! This was an interesting thing to discover; glad I brought it up."

The session ended with Michele's deep venture on that thought. As she walked away I wondered if I had fetched too much insight; I often struggled with to know how much was too much for clients to handle.

Process Notes: 23

Her new look seemed to have influenced her personality as well. Dressed in a crimson corduroy short skirt with brown knee-length leather boots, she looked like one of those rock-band artists along with her newly-coloured red hair. It is often amazing what our outer look can do to us internally. As she spoke, at the back of my mind was the image of how Michele was, a couple of months ago–shy, indecisive, anxious to disclose her identity often. The girl then and the one sitting in front of me this Friday weren't the same person! The contentment of witnessing clients grow through the therapeutic process was way more than the theoretical aspect of it.

I wondered where her concern for babies was emerging during the session since she was not keen on tying the knot any time soon. I confronted her about being dependent on others for her self-image and confidence. She understands the importance of being self-assured and independent, but fears standing up for her rights alone.

I was tired after completing her notes at the centre. Yet another

Friday and the first month of the New Year was gone. Was time really rushing that fast?

With the increased workload my desire to be lazy got accentuated. January and February were truly unforgiving in this regard. There were relentless submissions and deadlines with lots to cover within a short time. However, for me the internship was much more satisfying than writing papers.

The next Friday, I remember Michele acted unlike herself. It was quarter past four and there was no sign of her. I strolled to Rene's desk to check if Michele had left any message, which she had not. A soothing flute track relaxed my mind as I browsed through the internet. It was 15 minutes to five as per the clock stationed on the corner table. I knew for sure that Michele would not be coming. This was the first time that she missed a session without any prior information.

At that very instant I had the urge to call and check if things were fine with her but backed off. It was strange that I felt this way for her though many of my clients missed sessions without informing. Later I realized, it was probably because Michele had never done so before, and I was rather curious to know what had happened.

Occasionally there were cases when clients terminated without informing; though of course Michele's absence was not a sign of termination. Initially, I suffered from self-blame with many such clients, but later comprehended that it was they, and not me, who chose to shut down even before they had ventured in.

Walking back from the centre that evening, I felt maybe it was about time for Michele to move on. I had never imagined a single day's absence would make me think so profoundly. It was a mere non-attendance for a single session but thinking about it in depth threw up many more explanations. Her absence could have been an indication of striving for independence and separation from counselling. To a layman, I might sound a bit too peculiar but as far as counselling is concerned, nothing goes unattended. In fact, it is believed that each and every act of the client refers to some underlying meaning.

It was dark though there was an unusual whitish hue from the snow lying around since the snowfall on the previous day. I was getting used to the snow. I do not know if there is any correlation between our moods and nature; but whenever it snowed, I almost felt nostalgic. Maybe there was a connection, for me at least.

I changed the calendar that night after returning home. The new month, February, was the month of love. Love was in the air which was quite evident from the display of heart-shaped goodies and chocolate-coated strawberries to the pink-stuffed toys in the stores. The florist, whom I crossed every morning at the reservoir, displayed an array of fragrant roses. There was also something about the snow that made Valentine's Day celebration so special and romantic. My attention went towards some of the old couples exchanging sweet nothings and holding hands, as they strolled across the red-brick sidewalks. I found them to be more romantic than many of the young couples, who were rushing against time. Their romance seemed like an unexpected fresh breeze of innocence, even at that age, when mostly people start taking such relationships for granted. I wished someone special for myself as well with whom I could grow old.

Eventually I had made a lot of guy friends but there wasn't anyone special who I liked, as far as dating was concerned. Amanda had made special Valentine plans with her boyfriend. Teri and I decided to meet up and rejoice our single hood. Not that we were too excited for about it, but it was fun nonetheless. Monday morning during supervision, I discussed about Michele and my perspective to her queries. Sometimes, I wondered if she was ever confused about solving cases since suggestion of any client-related issues came so naturally and readily to her. I secretly wished I had those qualities that rendered her an expert in this field. Dr Sparks encouraged me to further explore and occasionally challenge Michele, sort of playing devil's advocate, to see if she was really prepared to face the outside world.

She suggested, "This is the most crucial stage in counselling when the client and the counsellor reach the transparency phase. A pseudo-questioning session is never a bad idea before facing everyone out there. This way she would at least be prepared with what to expect while discussing her sexual orientation with her family."

I spoke about Rupa's growing impatience as well and her husband's firm denial on external help even if it was professional. Dr. Sparks insisted on seeing Rupa personally during one of the sessions. I felt relieved that my supervisor took the matter in her stride.

Her suggestions gave me the confidence that I was on the right track. I had been seeing a lot of clients for the last 20 sessions or so and now they all were reaching a phase where they needed to take their own decision. The past couple of months had been an exploratory stage for most of my clients. Some even were planning termination, which I also discussed during supervision.

****

As Friday approached my work schedule became hectic.

Rupa showed up for her session and after a housekeeping discussion, I informed her about seeing Dr Sparks for an expert advice. Initially she was cross at my suggestion. Rupa returned to her natural skeptical attitude while reasoning why I asked her to do so.

Eventually I was able to convey my concern to her about her problem and that discussing it with Dr Sparks might open new avenues. Reluctantly, she agreed. We decided on fixing the appointment for next week.

Amidst other clients, I found myself becoming increasingly curious about what might have emerged last week that kept Michele away from the session. I was rather doubtful whether she would make it this week. I decided to call her this time, in case she missed this session too, to ascertain the reason. At the same time, I hoped that Michele would turn up and prove my assumption wrong, which was exactly what happened. I was undoubtedly delighted to see her at our usual 4 pm slot. My happiness must have reflected on my face which perhaps she had noticed too.

6 February, 2004

Session: 24

"You look very happy this evening!" Michele began.

I smiled and thought maybe it's because you showed up for the session. I said in return, "So, how have you been?"

Michele seemed somewhat inhibited compared to the other days. "Well, I have been just alright, busy and quite disheartened. However, before I say anything further, I really want to apologize for missing my session last week as I overslept. Generally, I finish classes by 3 o'clock, grab a quick snack, visit the library or loosen up with friends before visiting you. Last Friday, I felt unwell and decided to head back home for a quick nap before the session, and of course I missed it! I woke up only after quarter past seven!! My cellphone alarm ditched me. Sorry about the inconvenience."

To put her at ease, I added, "Well it happens! Thank you anyway for informing. So, what has been disheartening you?"

Instantly her face became gloomy. "That's what I'm keen on discussing." She continued, "Lately Rachael has been pestering me to initiate conversation about our relationship to my family. She wants to get settled soon after we graduate and get our respective jobs. She feels her family wouldn't mind accepting me, owing to their open-mindedness"

I knew this was too much pressure to cope with. "What is your take on this?"

Michele calmly stated her point, "I feel she's right, but I'm struck with fear! I want to disclose, but I can't gather enough courage to disclose."

I gently approached, "I do understand your dilemma. It's a tricky situation, but only you can solve it. Talk to Rachael and tell her that you would require some time to actually unveil all this to your parents. She might understand."

Michele seemed confused but remained silent. Her expression spoke enough, of being sandwiched between both sides.

"I'll talk to Rachael, but some day it has to happen and I really don't know how I'm going to do it. I don't know where and how to start!"

After a pause, she continued, staring at the floor, "I've just recently started getting along reasonably well with Mom during these past couple of visits, and am scared of losing it all again. I hope her counsellor has communicated the tenet, 'live and let live', to her. I hope Mom understands that it is a choice that makes me happy and is not a stigma on their status."

I asked, "I hope things work in your favour. Have you thought as to how you want to place it to them?" She had a brilliant suggestion to which I gave my full consent.

"I was thinking of writing to my parents, like a hand-written letter. It's personalized and Mom is fond of hand-written letters; something rare nowadays."

"I agree, it does add a personal touch; interesting!"

She continued, "Else, I could call and talk to Mom directly, though I am not sure what to say. Also, she might hang up on me without getting my point. However, on the flip side, conversing directly would allow me to know Mom's reaction right away instead of speculating about it."

"You've thought quite constructively about it. I like your assertiveness; whichever way you feel more comfortable, should be the one to be chosen," I suggested.

Michele smiled, "Thanks, I hope to maintain this courage. Maybe if I write, they would read my entire letter and I'll be able to suitably put my thoughts across."

I inquired, "Are you expressive and comfortable about writing?"

My question guided Michele to think more clearly. "I've never done such a thing before, but I do like to write. Talking, though, would be more feasible as I'll be able to articulate my feelings well, but I doubt if they'll listen. On the contrary, in the letter she can't switch me off."

"Looks like you almost answered your query while expressing these thoughts."

She was clever enough to know what I was hinting at. "Yes I did! That's the reason I like to think aloud here. I'm able to see things in perspective without any deception."

I felt her surging anxiety underneath my own skin. This is it, this is it!! She's almost there. I thought momentarily.

"If I direct you, it would be like spoon-feeding, without you gaining any insight. So, don't rush, think it over and do what feels right to you.

She responded instantly, "I'd like to write. It'll give me time to rephrase my feelings well and I'll not be questioned face to face for explanations."

I already saw the determination in her looks.

"Well, that makes me feel better now!" she chuckled.

"Would you be working on a draft or mentally revising before actually finalizing it?," I urged.

She filled in almost instantaneously, "Yeah! Maybe I'll initiate by referring about Rachael and how we were friends previously. Then talk about our relationship as partners and so forth. I think a draft would be helpful."

"Sounds like a plan," I said encouragingly. "Feel free to call in case you need to talk. I'm sure your parents will accept that same-sex relationships are no longer a taboo. It has been even legalized in some states now. They must understand this won't undermine your respect as an individual in society."

She listened carefully as if gaining knowledge about such facts.

After we ended the session, I revisited the session mentally. She made me proud today! This session marked one of the most meaningful moments ever since I joined Simmons.

I was relieved Michele was thinking practically about "coming out" to her parents. However, she thought it was all happening too soon and also that she was too young for a serious commitment. It seemed Rachael was acting as a catalyst to make Michele think on realistic terms. Although counselling did endow her with a lot of confidence, it was largely a consequence of her mother's changed behaviour towards her, but she fears losing her treasured love again.

Her openness to transform and resilience to keep going enables her to handle situations that are not easy to handle otherwise. Michele seems to have realized that homosexuality is just another identity, as her other identities like being a Catholic and Caucasian. It was time to let go off all her inhibitions, I thought.

****

Saturday morning I was all geared up to proceed with the pending work and later sneak out for a bit of fun. It was windy and more chilly than usual. The wind chime at the front door sang incessantly, swinging to the rhythm of the morning breeze; it was melodious. The sun was lurking somewhere behind the evergreens. The snow that was piled in Patty's backyard glistened weakly. I was preparing for the day with a cup of black coffee. The aroma filled my room; it was exactly what I required to feel rejuvenated. At 10 I started working on my paper which I completed past noon. I was tired and took a nap.

Later in the evening, Patty asked me to accompany her to the nearby grocer's, which I eagerly accepted. I picked up a few items as well which I thought would be required over the week; it saved me an extra trip to the grocer.

Patty, on the contrary, shopped like a typical American, buying almost everything on the shelves and her trolley was piled high. Most of them shopped that way, picking up things that was not required nor consumed.

In the forthcoming week, the weather conditions worsened making it impossible to step outdoors. A blizzard occurred on Tuesday as predicted and it swept the entire city with hail and snow. It was beyond my imagination that something as light and as pretty as snow could become so destructive. People missed work; schools, and almost all colleges, including Boston College and Simmons, had shut down, the train service was rendered slow due to the heavy snowfall on the tracks, and it took some heavy shovelling to control the condition. I stepped outside the following morning for a brisk walk but it was freezing cold. I was standing on the porch and before I knew my fingers had gone numb inside the gloves. I quickly rushed inside.

A few daring neighbourhood kids ventured outside to make snowmen and snowballs but they could not withstand the cold for long and slipped back in. I watched the street from the window of my room, not a single soul was to be seen outside, everything was frozen–from tree tops to rooftops. The park situated in front of Patty's house had been transformed into a snowfield. It would have been hard to know where the park ended and the road began had there been no fences. There were sporadic spells of hail as well, although the intensity was less than the previous evening.

Although the blizzard, which was a first-time experience for me, rendered us house-bound with its ferocity, it was actually fun to get some days off. What a perfect time to snuggle up and enjoy hot coffee, mocha or hot chocolate! Undoubtedly it was rather romantic outside provided one had the right companion.

Daniel visited Patty from New Hampshire every week. Looking at the bad weather though, he extended his stay with us. Patty was excited that she got to spend some more time with him as she often missed him during the weekdays. It was interesting the way they behaved like husband and wife, but were actually dating. Daniel was so caring that he took the daughters out during weekends to shop or to run necessary errands. Symphony and Courtney weren't much fond of him as he was of them. Owing to their mother's fondness they remained neutral in their behaviour towards Daniel. Patty was waiting for her daughters to graduate from school before marrying Daniel. She wanted to avail the single parents' grant aided by the State for her daughters.

Gradually the weather got better and now there was no reason to stay indoors anymore and soon things normalized. There was the sun back again, struggling to shine and spread some warmth, which was more than welcome. The trains functioned as per schedules and roads were cleared of the snow, though they became even more slippery from the accumulated ice resulting from the partial melting of the snow. I remember it being sunny after almost a week that Friday. People charged out of their houses gleefully to enjoy the brightness. It was freezing but dry, and a pair of warm mittens, coat, snow shoes and a hat were the perfect accoutrements required for enjoying the day. The varied moods of the weather and our own reactions to them were indicative of the resilience of human nature; something that I believe.

****

An Unexpected Surprise

They met, they connected,
they departed, but the memories remain forever

Dr Sparks was again away for a seminar depriving me of her weekly supervision following the week after the blizzard. I had no choice but to clarify some of my doubts during our group supervision with Dr. Sheri Ettenger, our group supervisor.

Dr. Ettenger, was in her late 30's, came across as a very bubbly person. She was full of new suggestions and always understanding what the interns felt before we mentioned. She spoke fast and I liked the way she expressed thoughts with endless examples from everyday life. Her staple breakfast which she often had at the centre due to lack of time would be milk and cereal with granola or strawberries.

The consecutive absence of Dr Sparks made me realize about the attachment I had developed for her unbeknown to me. She was the seniormost staff member and the head of the centre; her vast experience made her the best person to consult. Dr Sparks was nearly in her seventies, blonde, American, divorced and a professional whereas I was in my twenties, Indian and a fledgling counsellor. Was there anything in common? Superficially, there did not seem to be anything–but on a deeper level there certainly was; it was our passion for the profession. We exchanged professional experiences; Dr Sparks shared hers to enlighten me and I did the same to gain further insight. Words are inadequate to describe the relationship. She was definitely an inspiration to me.

During the initial phase, Dr Sparks guided me immensely regarding my way of being a "professional" within my approach, issues about culture shock and managing my unknown fears and worries during sessions. I do not know if other interns felt the same about her, but I knew I would not have been able to handle clients that efficiently if it were not for her. Maybe it was the warmth of her smile, her understanding demeanour or her interpretation that reassured me. I wondered if my clients found me that approachable. I would not have realized all this if she had not been away for a while.

I was aware that my days with her were numbered, just as they were with my clients. In the interest of time and to allot myself space for such changes, I decided to discuss terminations and endings with her in the forthcoming supervision. It was something I was aware of from day one, but my affinity with the centre was growing stronger with each successive day. The relentless cold and snow continued as usual and so much so that I stopped going out for a stroll. During these days I hardly saw Patty's family due to my chaotic schedule except on weekends. It was crazily busy! The course was really heavy, especially since I had opted for 12 credits that semester, which made it four courses. Generally three were a handful to manage, but in order to complete the programme soon, I took an extra course. Though it was a lot of extra hours of work, the end result I knew was worth the effort.

Throughout the week and the mornings remained dull and white from the snow accumulated all around. During afternoons, a sudden hint of sun sometimes made all things bright and beautiful.

On Friday morning the weather was getting gloomier progressively along with mild snowfall. I reached the centre at 8 am sharp, walking through the freezing icy path. A cup of steaming hot herbal tea got my numb nerves functioning back to somewhat normal. The internal heating system felt so good after facing the minus degree temperature outside. By now I had adapted to dress in layers according to the changing weather conditions. My long black wool coat looked beautiful with the snowflakes making a pattern all over it.

At the centre, the attendance of clients was low owing to the approaching finals and also perhaps due to the weather. There were very few who would leave the comfort of the heater and brave the freezing temperature to come to the centre to talk therapy. However, Michele was one of the very few who did brave the weather to keep her appointment. Rupa though missed hers.

I thought she must have become anxious about seeing Dr. Sparks and hence called off her session. She was unaware that Dr. Sparks was out for an urgent seminar. Another interesting fact was that she never called to cancel her appointments; it was as if I would assume her absence without any prior information.

13 February, 2004

Session: 25

In line with the previous session, we continued exploring more on Michele's fears regarding ""coming out". Besides, I also lightly touched upon Rachael's willingness to spend some more time dating and getting to know their mutual compatibility.

Michele agreed that it was indeed a big step to give in so early in a relationship. I was relieved. "Maybe you are right, I should talk to Rachael about dating a couple of months more; that way we'd get to know each other better. I'm hoping she wouldn't mind! Tomorrow after our special little celebration for the Valentine's, I'll talk to her. She'd agree in that romantic mood."

"I am looking forward to hear more on that, hope you enjoy your time together! Moreover, there's no harm in giving yourself some more time before settling in," I added.

There was a deep sigh before she spoke again, "As of now my only concern is telling my parents."

I nodded.

She took over, "Definitely they wouldn't be happy about it. Maybe Mom will get furious or coldly disown my existence in the family."

I interrupted, "Why do you always think about the negative outcome? I think after therapy your mother has become more open and respectful towards understanding you."

"Yeah, her changed attitude is the prime reason I'm even considering telling her. I know they'll get the shock of their life. Dad might revert to his drinking habit, which he left years ago. I feel guilty for adding all this stress in their lives."

"Well I don't think liking a same-sex person is wrong. You need to get out of this negative self-blaming attitude," I said firmly. "What about Emily? Can she help in anyway to convince them?"

"Emily will be away for her undergrad programme; it would have been great had she been there. I don't know when she's going to come home. It's better I rule her out as of now. I also fear facing Mom and Dad after they've read my letter. Wish I could simply run away!" Michele exclaimed.

I said supportively, "I'm proud of you the way you are facing this situation."

"I am hoping for something positive but I fear the worst!" Michele shrugged her shoulders while making the statement.

Michele paused to drink water from her bottle before resuming, "I wanted to share something else not related to this topic."

"Which is?," I asked, raising my eyebrows.

"I'm not sure if you are aware that soon I'd be starting my internship," she began.

I wondered curiously if she was referring to termination as she continued, "So you know once that starts, I doubt if our sessions could continue any longer. I mean most of my classmates have been allotted their respective sites already, but I haven't heard of mine as yet. I'm excited for it to happen; it has been my long-cherished dream to assist in the nursing department. Nonetheless, I feel extremely sad thinking about missing sessions."

"Well congratulations! Good for you, sounds interesting. Yes, terminations are disheartening for both clients and counsellors, especially with dedicated clients like you. There isn't much we can do about it; rather we should welcome the positive change. Feel free to call here anytime, as long as I'm at Simmons. I'm sure you'll get the site of your choice," I said.

"I'm hoping the same," she seemed sad though.

Without wasting much time I began, "Since there isn't much time left, we could start reflecting on termination and maybe on some future plans or anything else that you may wish to share before closing."

She spoke while wiping the tears from her eyes, "It would be really hard for me to not have this time. Counselling has always encouraged me, propped me up wherever I thought I'd fail. I terminated with Lisa last year but somehow it never felt so depressing. I wish I could change my internship timings and attend the sessions here as well."

Instead I reassured her, "Don't feel upset about missing sessions. Like I mentioned before, I am accessible through email or phone until the end of this semester. Alternately you can always sign up for a special appointment in my free slots and we could talk."

Michele said nothing but smiled appreciatively.

As I was wrapping up the session I inquired, "Would you be coming next week?" She confirmed, nodding vigourously, "Yes, of course! I can't afford to miss our last chance to meet."

Once the session ended, my mind kept wandering back to the first time I had met her and how things had evolved over the months, contributing to our relationship. From a counsellor's perspective, I evaluated myself whether I had been fair to her and had succeeded in guiding her empathetically and impartially without being judgmental. Had therapy been like a mirror where she could reflect on her real self fearlessly?

I stayed back in my office for some time with my thoughts. I was happy for Michele; at the same time I felt sad too. I felt a lump in my throat and a tear rolled across my left cheek, but I controlled myself. I knew this was inevitable, but never expected it so soon, that too, with one of my favourite clients. Michele was quiet during the time we discussed termination as her eyes filled up with tears. I wondered if the intensity of her sadness was beginning to turn into a mild depression. To pull her out of this state of mind, I restrained my own sadness during the session. My heart felt heavy and I knew I was also crying inside, but professionally, I knew that termination was important and ought to happen sooner or later. The more realistically I accepted it, the better it was for both of us.

I wrote her process notes, probably the last but one. There was so much to reflect, but I could hardly pen down any insight. It was rather one of the most factual, precise process notes I had written so far. I surprised myself because my notes did not elaborate on either of our emotions; sometimes the mind processes better than words do.

The evening proceeded as usual into a cold, freezing night by the time I reached home. I felt as if someone had drained out all my feelings and emotions. I began thinking beyond Michele in my effort to detach myself and accept termination more professionally. There were about 12 other clients to terminate with and so I had to be strong.

To master the technique of detachment with clients was not easy. On one hand I was trying to detach myself from Michele, but actually became even more concerned when I realized that in the forthcoming months she might not even have a counsellor to whom she could speak. There was an intense desire to resolve all the issues with all my clients before termination.

I recall not doing much that evening after returning home. I just made myself a sandwich and went upstairs to my room. Mixed thoughts crossed my mind while I lay awake in my bed. All of them were not confined to work but a lot of other stuff.

I reflected upon my changes in life thus far. To be living in Boston, it was almost close to two years and how quickly this phase had gone by. My days in Delhi all that happened for good, and the future ahead, so many unattended questions arose. I wondered if I would continue living in Boston or settle in for returning back. It all seemed like a jumbled crossword puzzle and they went on whirling in my mind until I fell asleep.

****

The following week was unlike the usual ones. I needed a space to vent out and free my mind from all the ongoing stress and emotional build-up. There could not have been anyone better than my supervisor for such matters.

Friends could also have helped but since it was regarding my clients I preferred talking to her. Termination was beginning to become quite tough on me. I especially took an appointment to discuss the process of termination.

It was an amalgamation of detachment, sadness, insecurity, as well as concern for my clients. She understood my mixed state of mind and conceded it as quite natural during initial terminations. She shared her own early experiences which were somewhat similar. It was indeed beneficial when I heard she felt the same way. Instantly it acted like an approval to my feelings.

On Valentine's evening I and Teri decided to watch a comedy

movie and later pamper ourselves with some treat. The movie was hilarious and we had a great time munching on those buttered popcorns loaded with calories. We chose a Thai restaurant for dinner. Most of the tables were either occupied or reserved for two. They had decorated the place with red heart-shaped balloons and pillar candles. Due to the long waiting time we dropped the idea. Instead we enjoyed the street foods and tit-bit snacks on Beacon Street. It was great a great walk through Beacon Street to Commonwealth Avenue after dusk. All the streets were lit up and one could feel the love spreading all around, especially while watching couples having a grand time together.

Unlike India, Valentine's Day in the US was not just meant for couples. People bought Valentine cards and gifts to even wish their parents, siblings and friends. Patty also presented me a sleek red bracelet for Valentine's Day. It was very sweet of her and I was not expecting it. I returned her warm gesture by bringing a bouquet of Orchids for the family. I knew Patty loved the violet ones.

It was past Valentine's Day and most of the celebrations were over. People were getting back to work and regular routine. The big sale for Patrick's Day and Easter was far off. I desperately needed to do some shopping but there was no time. The weekends were packed with pending work, household chores and socializing with friends; and during weekdays I barely had time to see the clock! In a way I was happy being busy; at least there was no time to miss my family. Wednesdays and Thursdays I saw a couple of clients and attended late-evening classes thereby returning home after 10 pm It was hard to stay awake on those nights to do assignments. At that time my favourite and most luxurious activity was catching forty winks.

Fridays were a bit relaxed as there were no classes and also it was close to the weekend. It was my favourite day of the week, but this Friday I felt a bit low due to terminations.

Soon after interns' discussion meeting, we headed to our respective offices. I had a feeling that Rupa would not show up this week also. I was bang on target about my hunch. It seemed she got scared about seeing Dr. Sparks and decided to discontinue abruptly. There were moments when I considered calling her but didn't. I wanted to give it another week's time. Often clients get intimidated by calls as if they are bound by the counselling relationship. They need to understand that it is their free will if they chose to come or not.

I wished that time would stop before three. I felt as if I was not prepared to deal with termination yet. I didn't know how it would be, what would I say to her, if she would actually see me again or get in touch next week? Although during supervision, Dr Sparks had elucidated upon such concerns, new questions began popping up. I knew it was nothing but nervousness because I am quite bad with goodbyes.

20 February, 2004

Session: 26

Michele looked pale and dull than usual. I wondered if it was termination or something else. It was one of those known moments when we both sat silently. I thought Michele was more experienced with termination as she had been through it once before–with Lisa.

I shifted my attention back to the session, to the present, and finally broke the silence. "This is probably the last time we share silence together. If I may ask, what has been occupying your mind all this while?"

Michele began weeping the very next moment. Her blue eyes were swimming in tears which spilled over and flowed down her cheeks. At that moment, I too failed to hold back my emotions and gave in to my tears. I never expected I would cry during termination. We remained silent. I felt somewhat embarrassed that I had given way to my emotions.

Clearing my throat quickly I stated, in an effort to get the session back on track, "Michele, I know it's hard but this is life. Partings are meant for new beginnings and the sooner you understand it, the better you'd feel. Also, I wouldn't like to see you all sad and tearful for the remaining forty-five minutes that we have. I want you to talk to me. This time is very precious for both of us and it might never happen again so why not make the best of it?"

Michele murmured, "I know! I agree to what you say, it makes perfect sense, but it is still so unacceptable! I can't believe that I won't be seeing you anymore."

I reiterated her thoughts in an optimistic way, "Let's look it this way; you can see me whenever you want as long as I'm at Simmons; and for now, you are taking leave due to your internship. Does that sound better?"

She only nodded, "Um…." Michele sighed gazing at the floor before continuing the conversation

"I've given two interviews last week and am just waiting to hear from them. One is the Newton Children's Hospital and the other one's in Cambridge. Let's see, I am keeping my fingers crossed and hoping for the best," she added, "These are the only two sites probable; if I don't make it there, then there aren't any back-up plans!"

"The waiting period can be quite draining," I responded while she continued anxiously.

"I've longed for this moment, hope I get it!" She smiled for the first time during that session, "I remember playing a nurse to my dolls when I was young and now all my dolls would be real people."

I encouraged her for the upcoming internship result. Michele then pulled out a piece of paper from her brown leather bag and said, "I have drafted something on what I would be writing to my parents. I know it's our last session, but can we discuss this for some time before closing?"

I was more than happy that she remembered to bring me a copy of her draft and warmly welcomed her suggestion, "Of course! I think it's brilliant that you thought of sharing it."

She handed the paper to me. Michele had a child-like handwriting though quite neat. The letter read:

"Dear Mom & Dad,

I have been thinking of letting you both 'in' my life for quite some time now. Ever since we have started seeing our respective counsellors, things have changed for the better, thank God. This will not be easy for you or for me, but I am still sharing because I have faith that both of you will accept and understand my point of view.

I have always been the so-called black sheep of the family, inferior to Emily in every way, be it studies, looks, or social skills. I never complained; time has healed all those wounds. During my childhood I often longed to ride my bicycle with Dad and cuddle in your lap Mom on murky winter afternoons. I heard my friends talk about vacations and outings with their parents; a dream still pending for me. I knew 'we' were different from 'them'. Emily often revolted against the restrictions you put on us, but I always appeased her saying 'Mom cares about us, so she teaches us good rules'. But I was not appreciated though I never questioned anything. I remember countless nights when Dad never returned home and Mom used to be terribly disturbed and behaved irrationally. I was naïve, scared and too young to understand the complexities. I remember slipping inside the quilt and hugging Emily in my arms on those dark nights. My pillow was my true friend; it never allowed the quarrels at daybreak to reach my ears. Mom's endless limitations on food often made me greedy for more. Thanksgiving had turned into a dreaded experience until the last one which was a breath of fresh air. Amidst all odds I survived.

I did not choose my past life but now I intend to choose my future. Living alone for quite some time now, I have discovered myself in new ways. I know you both will probably despise my next few lines, but I plead for your support.

I have had many off-and-on relationships in these past two years, most are known to Emily. Among them, some have been with girls. Is that surprising? It was surprising for me too when I first started dating them. However, the truth is I really feel more comfortable with women partners. Mom, I hope you will not disown me after reading this. I have had other same-sex relationships before but they were all short-lived, unlike my present one. Please do not stop reading until you reach the end of this letter. I hope you remember Rachael, the girl who visited me and whom you accused, knowing that she was a lesbian. Much to your surprise, she is the one who has stood by me at all times. Rachael loves me without attempting to change the person I am and undoubtedly she is the one with whom I wish to share my future. I have slept with her but that is not the sole reason for loving her. We share a bond that has not been there with anyone, not even both of you! Do you wish this was not true? I too, wished it were not so, though now I am happy being the way I am and do not regret a bit for owning this identity. It belongs to me and I belong to it.

The good times we shared together in the last couple of months I visited, fetched me the courage to 'come out' to you. Mom, Dad, your daughter has lived life on your terms for years but now she is ready to spread her wings wide open to a world she calls her own. Being a lesbian is not shameful. I too have the same religion, feelings and emotions as you do.

Please do not let my hopes down and deny my existence in your lives. I might have grown old, but not old enough not to want to snuggle into your arms Mom or go fishing with you Dad.

I love you both not for what you did in the past, but for anticipating your positive acceptance of my new future.

Love, Michele."

It was intense, touchy and I was rendered speechless after reading her letter. Michele looked at me with inquiring eyes, waiting in anticipation for my response.

I expressed my sincere appreciation, "Your letter is a signature of your emotions, your desires, your regrets and your optimism. I liked the last part of your letter where you ended urging their support for a happy future ahead."

"Thanks for the feedback— it means a lot to me." She continued, "You know sharing my draft with you, as a second opinion, has heightened my confidence to write to them for real."

On inquiring when she planned to do so, Michele mentioned she would be posting the letter to her parents within a week or so. Michele then abruptly inquired, "Do you think they'll accept me?"

"I see no reason why they wouldn't! Had I been in their shoes I would have, but again these are too sensitive issues and individual perception plays a big role. A letter is a great way to begin, also, later it'll be easier for you to continue the conversation over phone while convincing them."

Michele paused momentarily before agreeing. It seemed she was unsure if they would actually be convinced and then spoke, "I would've loved to see you after telling my parents. I wish the internship timings didn't clash."

I settled her regret immediately by suggesting her to fix up an appointment conveniently during my free slots.

Michele's silence indicated that she was not proceeding willingly towards the new change. I interrupted her thoughts to inquire what was upsetting her. Michele continued her silence, and all had cheerfulness was lost once again.

Softly she murmured, "I was thinking about my first day at the centre with Lisa and then with you. Time has gone by so rapidly that it's hard to imagine myself sitting here for the last time. Surprisingly I'm not feeling insecure, which was the case when Lisa left. I think my journey with you has been more substantial because with Lisa I got myself acquainted with counselling more as a process, than myself.

With you I became more explicit about my own expectations from counselling."

I felt a concluding speech maybe appropriate because I had never done this before. I began by swallowing my awkwardness, "It's not just hard for you— I feel the same way. This is my first termination with a steady client and I never thought it would be you. I've witnessed a lot of optimism and confidence within you in the past few months with regard to your thoughts, taking responsibility for yourself and putting them into action. There were times when I confronted a lot to help you to go from uncertainty to assertive decision-making, but you'd agree it's worth every effort. It's not easy to put yourself 'out there' in front of all those questioning eyes, but you've done it. I want you to be comfortable with your sexual identity always, like you feel right now."

Michele appreciated my words.

I concluded, "I just wanted you to know that changes emerge throughout life, but everyone's not able to shape them to their advantage. I'm glad you've been able to and hopefully will continue to do so in future. It has been a wonderful experience knowing you, good luck!"

It was almost time to bid her goodbye I could not believe that was indeed our last session. Michele slipped out a card from her bag, as she stood up, and handed it to me. This was unexpected, but even more so was when I heard her say, "Can I hug you once? It's the warmth of our relationship that I want to carry with me as I walk out of this room today." I was taken aback; as she had once again left me speechless. I wanted to hug her too, for the first and the last time but it could have been deemed as unethical if I had initiated it.

I stood up–we moved closer. The distance between us was now less than our respective comfort zones. Michele hugged me gently, raising her hands and touching my shoulder blades. I smelled her usual deodorant, only now I was breathing through it, "Strong one," I thought. I wondered what she felt about me.

It was one of those pure moments of appreciation between a client and a counsellor. Our hugging was purely within the ethical limits. We both were in tears and smiling as well. I had suddenly become comfortable sharing my emotions and letting her know that she would be missed dearly.

Although throughout our sessions, I had focussed on the prime purpose of her therapy, "coming out" as a lesbian and being comfortable with her identity; today I thought it had all taken a different meaning. It was not just about her sexual orientation but also a space where she could define herself, believe in herself and rebuild those assets, which were absent previously which she has longed for.

Michele held my hand before she left, "Wish I'd known you more than a counsellor, we would have been great as friends."

She still had a couple of tears falling off her cheeks and some suspended on her eyelashes. I simply smiled without nodding or commenting. She let go off my hand and turned back towards the chair to pick up her belongings. Within a fraction of seconds, after thanking me once more, she walked out. This time I knew she had actually gone and it was for good.

Her departure made me think deeply. I was touched by her thoughtfulness of the card. At the same so many feelings raced my mind. I wrote the following in that week's updates for her.

Process Notes 26

The silence during the session today transported me back to the time when Michele talked about Lisa incessantly after every sentence, to which now I could relate as to how difficult it must have been for both of them. Simultaneously I wished, hoped and wondered if Michele had any thoughts about me.

Her letter to her parents, which she shared with me duly, spelled out her childhood pain and anguish, which she had suffered. In spite of all odds, it was astounding how positively she spoke about her relationship and her parents' approval. There was an underlying sense of optimism throughout the piece.

During termination it was energizing to hear her identify with the changes she had gone through. She also accepted being pointlessly shy and naïve in the past, which had only added to lack of expression and led to low self-esteem.

****

To many, especially those in this profession, hugging a client might come across as being unethical. However, I would differ from that opinion because as long as the client is comfortable and my gestures are not intrusive or embarrassing her and vice versa, it is not unprofessional. In this instance, it was termination and therefore it was a display of care and appreciation. It is also true that bonding creates the power to heal all wrongs.

****

Analyzing Termination

Intrinsic healing is self–rewarding

I stood there in the middle of the room not moving an inch from the position she had hugged me. It was only after Michele left, that I questioned myself if all this was for real. Unwittingly, I had given in to her wish without much hesitation, it was like self-discovery. Her last words, "Known you more than a counsellor," rang in my ears a million times. My heart was pounding fast, with infinite thoughts racing through my mind, recalling her words. I could not make sense of what she had meant exactly. Was it a sign for friendship extending beyond our formal relationship or was she interested to know more about me as a person?

I opened the card Michele had given me. The card was a printed sketch of two hands, one facing the palm side up and the other reaching out towards it with the palm side down.

Inscribed below was: "THANK YOU FOR ADDING MEANING TO MY LIFE."

Michele had addressed my name inside the card on the top left-hand side, below which she wrote a message:

"My journey with you, thus far, has been quite self-replenishing. The subtle changes that I am beginning to make in my life promises me a hopeful future. I feel worthy of my identity now. I wish I could have shared my journey of life with you forever, but all prayers are not granted! Thank you for believing in me and enabling me with a space which I now define as my own.

Love always, Michele"

I found myself becoming extremely emotional after reading her card. This was my first acknowledgment card from any client. Michele's thoughtfulness and urge to feel connected reflected through her words. I regretted not reading it in her presence so that I could have thanked her in person.

I looked at my watch, it was close to six. It was not dark but there was a weak light which I could see from the window of my office which was on the fourth floor.

The cottony pale clouds, the trees, all looked pretty as ever. On the ground, students clustered in groups in front of the entrance, some were in the parking lot and few were making their way towards the other buildings or the main road. I had watched these activities a numerous times before, but at that time everything seemed unfamiliar or rather I was looking at everything with a different frame of mind.

Life goes on and always will no matter what. The presence or absence of a person does change it. I wondered how others dealt with termination. My emotions were muddled up together, I felt sad, hopeful, happy, and surprised, all at once. In spite of terminating, I was happy for Michele and a true sense of satisfaction surged through me.

I noticed Michele's self-reflection, as she introspected, and her inner strength which was the guiding light towards becoming the person she always wished to be. Sometimes pressures from the society curbs our individuality. Some ignore them, while others rebel and achieve their goal of establishing their identity. Michele had learnt the hard way but she had succeeded.

It was true that bringing a smile, optimism and adding meaning to others' life was very satisfying. It was the kind of contentment, which made feel great about counselling. It is true that realization often occurs after the act itself and this was true for me as well. As long as she was there, she was my sincere client. It was only after her termination that I realized that she had been like a teacher to me, who challenged my capabilities to delve deeper into the fundamentals of counselling homosexuals. The profound meaning attached to counselling only came to light post my first termination.

I walked outside towards the helpdesk and noticing me arrive, Rene murmured, "How did the last session with Michele go?"

I knew Rene was aware it was her last session, however since I was not in a mood for conversation; I simply smiled and nodded to affirm that it was satisfying. Rene was a fairly soft-spoken person with whom I often confided regarding clients, hectic schedules and occasionally my personal matters as well, but today I did not feel like talking much.

I left the centre alone that evening as Lesley was still tied up with her client. Settling inside the train, I thought of two individuals who met, achieved a purpose and a strong bond and parted. They knew they would never meet again. Time would erase their connection like footsteps in the desert sand. It was Michele and I that I was thinking about, maybe it should have been easy to 'let go' as I was aware that this was an integral part of counselling, but a world of other factors had also shaped our professional relationship.

****

My day started with supervision with Dr Sparks, it was a much-awaited one as I had a lot to fill in about the past week. There was a lot to share, which included whereabouts of old and new clients, treatment plans, the approaching terminations and, of course, about the one who terminated.

Dr Sparks patiently attended to updates on various issues. I informed her about Rupa's continued absence. It struck me that she might have even terminated silently because coming would mean meeting the supervisor. "I wonder what the big fuss about seeing you is," I exclaimed to her.

She smiled her usual suspicious way and continued her silence. It was only during the course of our conversation that she mentioned, "Clients sometimes refrain from becoming the centre of attention. It makes them feel even more vulnerable. Rupa might have felt the same way, I guess."

I agreed with her view. Probably that might have been the reason. I spoke about Michele last because I knew it would take more time than the other matters and thus clarified all other queries prior to starting on that topic. Interestingly, the only question that Dr Sparks asked was if I was comfortable when Michele asked if she could hug me. I affirmed that it was a warm gesture which I welcomed, and shared my true feelings, without hesitating even for a minute. Initially, I felt Dr Sparks was rather surprised with my accepting openness. Later in the conversation, I expressed my appreciation for Michele for her spontaneity with which she embraced our relationship.

Michele's remark before she left, about knowing me more than a counsellor, was also discussed. Dr Sparks chuckled hearing this and I sensed she was somewhat taken aback.

"Did she actually say that?," she exclaimed, a bit louder than her usual tone.

Generally it was hard, almost impossible to surprise her; it seemed her age and experience had been through permutation-combination of most situations, but this time she stared back at me through her bifocal glasses with a little astonishment.

We deliberated for while and finally she suggested, "I feel Michele had become quite emotionally attached to you, and therefore sensed a gap, imagining your absence. She might have wished you both were friends. She certainly wasn't curious to know about your personal life. Sometimes, clients fall in love with their counsellors unknowingly, something like transference, but that can only be known if they admit it explicitly. In your case, I would just keep it as 'urge-to-be-friends'."

I never thought Michele would ever feel that close to me to carry a casual friendship further. I felt both honoured and thrilled, at the same time.

The general reaction of the clients during termination was mostly sad, with exception of some like Beth, who had better reasons to terminate. I inquired about dealing with these moments.

Dr Sparks suggested that it was quite natural for clients to feel depressed prior to termination and fear losing all therapeutic contact. In some cases, they even wish they could replace their partners with their counsellors. She laughed about it lightly, but I did not find it amusing, maybe because it was the first time I had heard of such a thing. The supervision session proved extremely beneficial, particularly knowing facts about termination.

The following Friday, I had two empty slots, Rupa's and Michele's. There was no schedule with a new client either. It felt strange because I had grown fond of both of them over the course of our interaction. I thought about them and their probable conditions.

Time and again I found myself becoming concerned about Rupa's well being and if she had settled her differences with her husband. It would sound more like an intrusion if I called now; I thought she preferred the silence. Hence, I controlled my urge to call her.

During Michele's time-slot, I missed her presence in the room. I wished she had called to inform about her parents' reaction on receiving her letter.

This room had witnessed so many ups and downs, fears, happiness, and surprises of my clients. It had witnessed millions of moments within hours of sessions. I thought this had become a place where one could simply emote effortlessly, such a cathartic thing to do. Interestingly, many a times, I had my personal counselling sessions with Dr. Sparks in my office as well, due to lack of availability of rooms. I knew I would miss this room once I left Simmons and it would hold a very special place in my memories for a long time to come.

Holistically, all my experiences at the counselling centre had proclaimed insightfulness, not just to my professional growth, but also personal relationships. My initial reluctance to reveal personal feelings and rigidity of thoughts to disclose about myself made me miss out on the core of connecting with clients. Gradually, as this was sorted out, I began disclosing my thoughts and insights with clients. I became less self-conscious. In addition, sharing a close empathic relationship with clients also instilled a lot of confidence in me.

I would call myself quite an impatient person in general, but the counselling programme along with my clients taught me to become more patient. I began to realize that hasty decision-making often worsens the situation, but analyzing the process or thoughts lead to better solutions.

Healing or counselling, as it is said, is a process that affects both parties— the healer and the one to be healed. Similarly, I got healed, in the process of connecting with my clients. It was not just professional; I could feel such changes occurring also at a personal level.

More so, it would not be wrong to admit that Michele was among the first to acquaint me with the LGBT community and their ongoing struggle, which contributed immensely towards a sensitized growth. I got relatively familiarized with the type of embarrassment, fear and shame they often underwent for belonging to the LGBT group. Interestingly, it became more comfortable with time to deal with such clients than the other interns. I especially became quite receptive to the emotional needs of those who had not "come out" yet.

As I belonged to the Indian community, a minority in the

US, clients felt less inhibited to disclose their humiliations and so forth, maybe because many regarded me as being one of them, in terms of encountering differential treatment–in my case because of my ethnicity.

This process of acquainting myself with the LGBT community, along with Dr Spark's supervision, enabled me to identify my own emotions and recognize the intent behind them and most importantly, to detach from my own emotions and be able to step into my clients' shoes and empathize with their mental state. For instance, in spite of feeling gloomy because of my personal matters on some days, I was able to rejoice in the success of my clients. This ability to detach from myself and feel the clients' emotions was a major step in my professional learning. Besides, I learnt various aspects about life from my clients' experiences. It was like witnessing different shades of life under one roof. Looking back now, I realize and accept that it is absolutely impossible to empathize with others without being affected or going through some process within ourselves, the way I experienced it.

Days rushed by like the speed of light. I was loaded with work and other clients. Most of them were Americans with the single exception of Japanese, who initially was quite challenging since she neither spoke nor understood English. Apart from communicating through her translator, we worked a lot through sign language and drawings. This was new to me and pleasantly enlightening. It only made me realize that compassion, empathy and understanding was not hemmed in by language. Amidst all clients and despite my busy work schedule I did not fail to think of Michele quiet often.

I thought of her the most while dealing with clients who were undergoing similar lesbian issues. Her pronounced optimism and struggle to carve an identity of her own always inspired me. In retrospect, she endowed me a brilliant opportunity to learn about life from a different perspective. My presence was more like a mirror, where she could reflect and see her real self, uninhibited.

The more I thought about Michele, the more I appreciated her. It was fascinating to see what emerged out of one's true self-image, which sometimes was the opposite of what she portrayed initially. I learnt that allowing this space to clients for exploring their self-image is the core of therapeutic healing.

During off hours, when we sat together at the cafeteria Amanda and Teri too mentioned feeling the same stress due to terminations at their respective internship sites. It was tough to remain detached at a level where one would go unaffected by the clients' feelings. The days had passed with such urgency that none of us realized how fast the time was ending.

I mostly reached home late due to completion of a lot of paper work for those clients who had terminated. All the interns were needed to submit their complete files, which took quite long to get assembled. Patty would be awake some days to answer the door for me, or else I had an extra key. I hardly got to catch up with the family or Shelby, my roommate. My course was so consuming that it extracted all the energy out of me.

Time was changing and so was the season. There was less of snowfall and more of snow turning into slit, making it a slippery mess everywhere on the roads. Of course, I felt the cold had gotten bitter because when the snow melted it became way chillier than the snowfall. The locals of Boston were accustomed to all this but newcomers like me often slipped walking on the hilly slit tracks.

****

A Memorable Ending

The sky is the darkest before dawn,
endings are signatures of new beginnings

A couple of days later I heard from Michele while counselling another client. We could not converse for long as I was in session, but promised to return her call soon. Michele's voice sounded so familiar on the phone even after a fortnight's gap; I was pleasantly surprised! I could not wait to hear from her and how things were going at her end. Soon after ending my session, I shut the door and dialled Michele's cellphone.

She updated me with her latest internship schedule, which obviously clashed with her session timings, as she had correctly predicted. I inquired if she wanted to talk about anything in particular, to which she informed in about her parents' response. I attended to her conscientiously.

Her parents had undergone tremendous mental turmoil after reading her letter. Further she tearfully continued, "Mom was literally in a shambles, realizing that Rachael is my partner. She felt betrayed and ashamed."

In course of our conversation, she also declared confronting her parents to let her breath and live the way she wanted. Though things did not sound much in her favour, I found Michele quite calm and poised compared to when she was being counselled. Finally after many agitated conversations Michele had given up persuading them. She felt time would be the best healer to bridge the communication gap that had been created after revealing the truth. Not only did they refuse to talk to her from then on, but also asked Emily to do the same. Towards the end of our conversation, Michele stated that recalling insights from our sessions gave her the courage to go on despite all odds. She was hopeful that things would improve with her parents some day and they would accept, support and love her just the way she wished and hoped.

Unexpectedly, I felt better and actually refreshed after that telephonic conversation with Michele. I knew she had grown up to my expectations, of what I had envisioned of her.

My parents were far removed from the world of counselling, Dr. Sparks was out of town on work and so was Dr. Sheri and, ethically, I was not allowed to discuss cases with my frineds, so I shared this experience of contentment with myself. A smile, memories of the time Michele started, some doodles of "happy faces" with remarks on my notepad and a cup of hot jasmine tea was my celebration to commemorate the moment. I knew there was a long way to go before she could unite with her family, but her attempt to deal with it optimistically was reason enough to rejoice. Michele has been one of my most successful clients, reaching out to the world from the cocoon with her astounding self-confidence.

Michele kept me updated now and then about her whereabouts and her life through emails and phone calls. Once, I remember, she called to share how certain she had become more comfortable with Rachael and their progressing compatibility. Most of her worries and anxieties, which included her internship, as well as the stagnated relationship with her parents, found expression through her emails. She was better at writing than articulating over the phone. I replied to her doubts as and when needed, Michele was one of my only clients who kept in touch even after she formally terminated.

Towards the end of March, her calls became sporadic, as she got busy with her internship. By then it had been quite some time she had been out of therapy. By now she had learned to deal with various issues, take decisions with initiative, with or without counselling, I thought of it as very encouraging, and accepted it that every good thing comes to an end, so did this. I knew Michele had become quite adept at handling issues sanguinely. Time faded our connection; I thought of her occasionally and hoped well for her.

Interestingly, I never thought of her as anyone different just because she was a lesbian. Initially, yes I was skeptical but as I knew her better I realized how wrong I was. Her concerns mostly revolved around relationship issues, but that never became the soul of knowing her as a person. It was my overall interaction that evolved into a professional liking for this client, a feeling I shared for many of my clients.

Being eloquent with a lesbian woman was like a kiss of hope, especially for all those who are sailing in the same boat and wish to "come out" to the society. Their aspirations, hopes, wishes and desires are no less or different than straight people.

Owing to our respective busy lives and commitments, we both drifted apart. We no longer spoke to each other; also my internship was coming to a close. I had become adept in terminating with clients and as did many of my classmates and interns at Simmons. Interestingly, it was not as nerve-wrecking with others as it was with Michele, though emotionally it was still draining. Some presented me with tokens of remembrance, cards, and so forth. In the beginning it hurt, but as I terminated with more and more clients, I realized it became more of a professional formality. There was no choice but to terminate with all of them, as I was coming to the end of my internship, which took away the sensitiveness of the situation.

There were different reactions from different clients; some took it sportingly, some wept, some thought of it as an opportunity to confess, while some remained indifferent and did not express their feelings. It was almost within two to three weeks when I wound up all terminations. Intermittently, I thought of Michele and thought of how different she was. I was glad I had clients with whom I had a bonding that was more meaningful than just conducting sessions, completing paper work, and analyzing perspectives.

Years later I still think of all my clients and I wonder how their lives might have changed for good. Did Michele finally settle down with Rachael or was she dating someone else? I wonder if her parents had finally accepted her. Above all, I selfishly imagined if any of them ever thought of me, especially Michele. It has been long since I saw her last, but I still cared for her not only as a client, but also for the person she was.

****

After returning to India, I became acquainted to many interesting changes with the increased influence of Western culture, merging with our own traditions. I realized, in spite of such westernization, we, Indians, often held back discussing issues such as sexuality or one's partner preference.

Even today, sadly enough, a vast majority of people are under denial and openly ridicule the gay/lesbian population. Though this community undergoes rejection in the US as well, in India it is far more pronounced. I actually came across people who thought of homosexuality or the slightest inclination of being a gay, lesbian or bisexual as a disease which could be 'treated' with medication.

We may have become 'modern' in many areas today, but within our modern society, there are countless diminutive gestures, expressions, impulsive reactions that are directed towards differential behaviour, especially towards the sexual minorities, which are indicative of our inhibitions. It seems much like a mental block that in spite of the tremendous exposure to other cultures and influences through the internet and the media, we are rigid about accepting realities of life. It is not that such issues pertaining to homosexuality only happens in the West, there is as much prevalence in India as well. Not bringing forth such issues only reflects our ignorance towards reality, and probably that is the reason a lot of gays/lesbians/bisexuals fear "coming out" to their loved ones. Under such conditions, the person often suffers from major depression or mental stress, which affects their overall well being and personality.

Personally I think that clients with such concerns need unconditional acceptance, love and support from their families as the first vital step towards opening up. Sexual orientation or partner preference of a person is only a part of his/her identity just as their other identities. Thus, under no condition should it impede the professional or personal growth of a person.

In the West too, parents often find it hard to accept such reality, but then the society gives them enough space and freedom to practice their choices. Those belonging to this community are fortunate to be born in the West; I sadly put this forth because I have not come across the same kind of flexibility to exercise one's choices without condemnation from society in India Some states in the US have even legalized gay marriage, which has taken care of issues of insurance coverage, inheritance and the like, concerns that are important in any long-term relationship. This is not to say that there is no opposition to homosexuality in the US.

India has a lot of contradictions, all existing simultaneously. While on one hand there is denial of homosexuality, there are liberal surrogacy laws which have made it possible for many homosexual couples to have children. However, the beneficiaries have been only foreign couples so far. This only underlines the fact that human beings are complex and it is their myriad differences that keeps social anthropologists occupied.

****

This book is created from my personal experiences and thoughts. I have been fortunate to be able to experience the best of both worlds. Looking back, I feel nostalgic about my memories of Boston. It has been years since I last heard from or saw Michele or any of my clients for that matter. Life moves on but it is only our memories that remain intact forever.

****